THE
MUSCLE TEST
HANDBOOK

FUNCTIONAL ASSESSMENT, MYOFASCIAL TRIGGER POINTS AND MERIDIAN RELATIONSHIPS

Hans Garten MD DIBAK DACNB DO (DAAO) FACFN

GUEST EDITOR FOR THE INTERNATIONAL EDITION
Joseph Shafer DC CCSP DIBAK

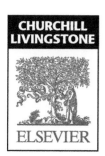

CHURCHILL LIVINGSTONE

ELSEVIER

Edinburgh   London   New York   Oxford   Philadelphia   St Louis   Sydney   Toronto   2013

CHURCHILL
LIVINGSTONE
ELSEVIER

First edition published in English © 2013, Elsevier Limited.
All rights reserved.
First edition published in German under the title *Das Muskeltestbuch*
First Edition 2007, © Elsevier GmBH, Urban & Fischer, Munchen

This edition of the Muscle Test Handbook by Hans Garten and
Joseph Shafer is published by arrangement with Elsevier GmBH,
Urban & Fischer Verlag, Munich

ISBN 9780702037399 (The Muscle Test Handbook)
ISBN 9783437583407 (Das Muskeltestbuch)

British Library Cataloguing in Publication Data
A catalogue record for this book is available from the British Library

Library of Congress Cataloging in Publication Data
A catalog record for this book is available from the Library of Congress

Notice
Neither the Publisher nor the Authors assume any responsibility for
any loss or injury and/or damage to persons or property arising out
of or related to any use of the material contained in this book. It is
the responsibility of the treating practitioner, relying on independent
expertise and knowledge of the patient, to determine the best treatment
and method of application for the patient.

The Publisher

your source for books,
journals and multimedia
in the health sciences

www.elsevierhealth.com

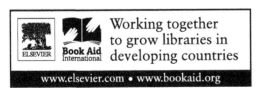

Working together
to grow libraries in
developing countries

www.elsevier.com • www.bookaid.org

The
publisher's
policy is to use
paper manufactured
from sustainable forests

Contents

Manual muscle testing is a functional neuromuscular assessment tool and should be considered an indispensible component of a modern clinical examination. Although its use is only now beginning to be widely appreciated, manual muscle testing has a relatively long history and was probably first introduced to physical medicine in the USA by Lovett and Martin (1916) followed by Kendall and Kendall (1952). Kendall's text is by far the most widely dispersed and it is this book that inspired George Goodheart to investigate the clinical merit of manual muscle testing. In Europe the muscle test has a much shorter history and Janda (1994) appears to have been the first to describe its varied clinical uses. Applied kinesiology (AK) muscle testing was already being taught and used in Europe by the time Janda published his text.

Janda's description of muscle testing differs somewhat from the earlier works yet both he and Kendall use a graduated system for the evaluation of muscle 'strength' capacity. Applied kinesiology (AK) is a term used to describe the manual muscle testing diagnostics primarily developed by Goodheart (1964). Goodheart took classic manual muscle testing and moulded it into a precise diagnostic tool. Prior to him, muscle testing was used primarily to diagnose motor nerve pathology and assess recovery during and following therapy. He astutely observed changes in muscle resistance patterns in the absence of motor nerve pathology. What he discovered was that disturbances anywhere in the body would lead to changes in normal muscle contraction patterns. The main and most notable change from the past was that the muscle test became less an assessment of contractile strength and more an assessment of proprioception, spinal and central nervous system regulation and the effects they have on neuromuscular function.

Strengthening a weakened muscle by exercise is only sensible and efficient if neuromuscular, proprioceptive control of the muscle is intact. Usually, it is not the loss of strength in a muscle that is most important, but a degrading of normal neuromuscular function both within and between individual muscles that is responsible for the greatest number of disturbances. AK is the only available method that allows for a clinical diagnosis of this type of dysfunction. This is simply and convincingly demonstrated when a normoreactive (strong) muscle is tested, followed by testing a hyporeactive (functionally weak) muscle. Because of this, AK muscle testing provides a fast and accurate functional assessment tool in sports medicine. In athletes even minor injuries causing subtle dysfunctions can mean the difference between winning and losing a competition.

AK offers an arsenal of therapies that can normalize muscles found to be functionally inhibited (hyporeactive) or conditionally over-facilitated (hyperreactive). Lesions to the origin and insertion, reactive muscle patterns, fascial shortening as well as other muscle dysfunctions originating outside the muscle structure (i.e. vertebral level of motor supply and the rest of the factors of the viscerosomatic system) can all be evaluated and treated using AK methods. There are a host of therapeutic options available within the AK arsenal. A detailed explanation of these therapies and their subsequent uses may be found in the *Neuromuscular Functional Assessment (NFA)* series by this author (at this printing available only in German) and in Walther's classical *Applied Kinesiology, Synopsis* (Walther 2000) or the flow chart manual by Leaf (1996).

This book was written with the intent to bring together two seemingly opposed parties. Practitioners of AK consider muscle inhibition the primary dysfunction and any hypertonic shortening a consequence of some other muscle inhibition. The other group consists of those who have traditionally focused on muscle hypertonicity as the primary dysfunction, aiming to 'relax' them. The truth, as is so often the case, seems to lie in the middle. There is an impressive wealth of therapeutic knowledge in normalizing the function of inhibited muscles to be found in professional applied kinesiology (PAK). Muscle energy techniques for the normalization of mainly hypertonic muscles stems from works in physical therapy and osteopathy. It should be obligatory that these two groups be combined into a more integrated therapeutic approach. Until a more profound understanding is in place, the question as to whether musculoskeletal problems are derived from a primary hypertonicity or as a consequence of a functionally inhibited antagonist, is less important.

First published in German, this text focuses on being a reference manual for the daily practice of orthopaedics, neurology, general medicine, physiotherapy, chiropractic and osteopathy. The English version has not altered this theme. The decision to translate it into English allows the manual to be more widely distributed to all of the above professions. Those who understand both German and English might note that the text has been changed slightly from the original German. It became evident that a direct translation did not manage to convey the exact intent found in the German edition. In some chapters the English narrative is a bit longer than that found in the German. Joseph Shafer is a colleague and Diplomate in AK. With many years of experience, he was chosen to make the corrections to the English version of the text. A simple translation could not be made and he spent innumerable hours refining the English translation. He is now considered a co-author of this edition.

Our many fruitful discussions have helped to improve the quality not only of this English version but also of its German equivalent.

I feel that I must also express my heartfelt gratitude to the alternative medicine division of the publisher. Their patience and willingness to make quality prevail, despite a tight budget and the long delay made by the decision to 'redesign' the entire English wording, makes a big company into a very personal entity. These are qualities which sometimes tend to get lost in this short-lived period of mankind's existence.

Hans Garten
2013

From the humble muscle test, Goodheart conceived and developed a whole new system of clinical diagnostics that only now is beginning to be fully appreciated. His astute observation of muscle resistance changes following structural dysfunction, disease states, nutritional deficiencies and emotional trauma, lead to what is now widely known as applied kinesiology or AK. Goodheart began teaching these principles in 1964. By 1970, a core group of 12 doctors, including Goodheart, founded the International College of Applied Kinesiology (ICAK) with the intent to further develop and document AK, as well as educate healthcare professionals. This discipline now encompasses a vast array of evaluation procedures and therapeutic techniques. Many of the techniques were directly developed within AK while others have been adapted into the sphere of AK and are taken from chiropractic, osteopathy, medicine and cutting edge scientific research.

Blessed with an almost photographic memory, Goodheart remained the primary developer of AK until his death in 2008. Not only was Goodheart a very fine physician but he loved winged flight and the feeling of sitting behind the wheel of a powerful car. He was a fighter pilot in World War 2 and even though he chose to continue chiropractic studies, the joy of flying remained with him throughout his life. This passion for flying is reflected in some of the classic techniques he developed in AK. The PRY-T or 'pitch, roll, yaw & tilt' technique and his reference to the hyoid bone as the 'gyroscopic' guiding device for the body, can both be attributed to his enthusiasm with flight.

In keeping with this line of thought, one might say that for AK, Goodheart was much like the first stage of a rocket lift-off from earth. He was the mighty power source without which the traditional gravitational bonds to clinical diagnosis could not have been overcome. His passing left AK with this wonderful panoramic view from where it had come but perhaps what is more important is that he left an even more astounding image of what lay ahead in that still undiscovered universe called the understanding of humankind. Goodheart's departure is as if the first stage of the rocket has been jettisoned and AK must now finely tune its orbit, establish a new equilibrium and decide on the direction to follow in the pursuit of further development.

The Goodheart years saw a fulminating AK expansion, with one new finding after another being discovered and one technique after another being developed. In some ways, like the proverbial double-edged sword, the enthusiasm for discovering new and exciting possibilities awaiting one around the next corner tended to leave earlier findings choking on the spent gases from the passing rocket. This has left the professional AK organization with very important responsibilities for the future. Probably the first and the most critical task is to validate, redefine and refine the art of manual muscle testing so that it can be learned and practiced in a standardized fashion. The second mission is that of fully comprehending and classifying the techniques already available within the discipline. The third is to continue to explore and uncover the vast potential still awaiting discovery within AK.

Early AK development was primarily made within the chiropractic profession. Very few outside the chiropractic profession knew of its existence. A medical psychiatrist, John Diamond, was fortunate and clever enough to understand the importance of what Goodheart was teaching from the very early years. He, alone, was one of the first health practitioners outside chiropractic to embrace the methods developed by Goodheart. A few dentists, like Harold Gelb, also realized the impact AK could have in physical diagnosis and began applying AK in their own professions. But it was not until the mid-1980s, when AK was beginning to gain interest in Europe, that other health professions became involved in a more serious way. The European development, other than the influence of Goodheart, is, without a doubt, the most fortuitous and significant event in the growth of AK. The extraction of AK from the homogenous thinking of the chiropractic profession has helped to expand AK into a truly multi-professional diagnostic system.

The accuracy of the muscle test is paramount to the final diagnostic success of the practitioner and this makes it both the key link and the weakest link in the analytic chain of events. Just as in the game of chess, the lowly muscle test, like the lowly pawn, is more often than not the predicator of just who will win in the end. Even though the accuracy of the muscle test was always stressed in the past, precision was often still lacking. Part of this is due to the fact that the art of muscle testing seemed to be simple and easily performed. Discrepancies and errors noted within the various books on the subject abounded, especially in those where 'kinesiology' muscle testing was described in more popular terms. An understanding of the nuances involved in AK muscle testing was often, in many instances, left wanting due to the natural ignorance of a young, developing profession. The overriding mystique surrounding AK where it is assumed that it is possible to diagnose everything from allergies and emotional states to Zen energy imbalances, quickly causes one to lose sight of the fact that all this is inherently dependent upon the accuracy of the muscle test.

The relative ease of use, combined with the fact that there is no need for a large investment in equipment, made AK the perfect avenue for a host of alternative therapies to show their validity and efficacy. The ubiquitous use of this 'quasi-AK' and its success in the new age culture caused the professional use to suffer terribly. Forms of this new age muscle testing exist to this day in various, somewhat dubious forms. One of its uses is to determine whether food in the supermarket is good to eat. Another more recent phenomenon is to sell fake armbands that supposedly improve balance, coordination and physical performance; all based on some kind of pre- and post- muscle test outcome.

Doctors and therapists, who used AK professionally, witnessed the trend to call all forms of muscle testing 'Kinesiology' and responded by trade-marking Professional Applied Kinesiology (PAK®), a term which must not be used by anyone not having fulfilled the educational criteria as defined by the ICAK.

In a strange quirk of events, the first widely published muscle testing manual was *Touch for Health* by John Thie. It quickly became a classic in the new age movement. Although fraught with many errors, it was one of the first attempts to describe the AK phenomenon and has remained a cult text to this day. The first professional text *Applied Kinesiology* by Walther followed shortly thereafter and its still valid successor, *Applied Kinesiology, Synopsis* (Walther 2000), remains in publication. They, as well, contain certain errors that are consistent with the understanding of AK muscle test at the time. Despite this, the texts by Walther are factual, historical descriptions of early AK development and methodology.

One of the first medical doctors to become involved in AK in Europe, Wolfgang Gerz, produced a very innovative pocket muscle testing manual. He should probably be best known, however, for urging Goodheart to accept a definition of what is probably the first logical diagram of how a muscle test is performed. To this day it is still used as the standard.

This book is a humble muscle test tribute to the legacy left by George Goodheart. The muscle test is the pawn upon which the diagnostic game is won or lost. In this text, Hans Garten has taken that next logical step in the direction of accepting one of the most pressing responsibilities for the future of AK – a return to the basic foundation from which AK was born, the specific and precise muscle test. No other component of AK is more important. Everything that is AK, and that will be AK in the future, rests upon the cornerstones formed by these tests. Based upon the classic muscle test, this book is the next generation in AK understanding of muscle testing.

Hans Garten, taking the knowledge from the past, has improved upon it and imparted an even more strict and extremely meticulous interpretation for executing each muscle testing procedure.

In addition to the classic AK muscle tests for detecting functional weakness, stretch tests and post isometric relaxation procedures for the hypertonic, shortened muscle are integrated. The latter are probably better known outside the spheres of AK and this volume thereby is an effort to bridge the gap between the various 'muscle working' professions.

There is no substitute for a 'hands on' learning experience and, ideally, this manual should be augmented by attending practical workshop sessions. There is a less well-known yet relevant phrase that states, 'Well begun is half done'. Stressing the need for high quality muscle testing, this text emphasizes that thinking. The student who learns the methods described within it will clearly have a solid base for further perfection in AK diagnosis and therapy.

Joe Shafer
2013

Manual muscle testing for motor function evaluation is indicated for all types of disorders, even following acute injury. It is also useful in almost any painful condition as well as for functional and degenerative diseases of the neuromuscular system. As a tool for evaluating 'subluxations' or 'fixations' of the vertebrae and for extremity joint disorders other than those of a primary inflammatory origin such as is found in rheumatoid arthritis, muscle testing is invaluable. When performing a functional, neurological examination the muscle test can be indispensable. Manual muscle testing may be considered a very specialized 'differentiated deep tendon reflex', as they both use the same neurological pathways. Muscle testing, however, provides more clinical information than solely reflex stimulation (muscle stretch reflex, myotonic reflex, see Ch. 12 in Garten 2012).

Primary and secondary muscle dysfunction

A direct injury to or local degenerative pathology of a muscle will disturb its internal neural circuitry. These may be categorized as a primary muscle dysfunction or 'intramuscular disorder'. On the other hand, should the local neuromuscular structure (proprioceptors, intra- and extrafusal fibres) be intact, muscle dysfunction may also be caused by disorders in the centrally modulated neuromuscular reflex circuit. These may be called secondary in nature (see motor function control, Ch. 12 in Garten 2012).

Most of the secondary disorders have origins in entrapments at the level of the intervertebral foramen, at peripheral entrapment sites or as a result of disorders in suprasegmental central control from the brain. Disturbances in central regulation may be due to many things, even those seemingly unrelated to the CNS. For example, any change in the sensory afferentation arriving from the periphery may have wide spread consequences in the central integrative state of the brain. These alterations will undoubtedly change motor function.

The viscerosomatic reflex phenomenon is well-established and accepted scientifically. Muscle–organ associations, on the other hand, are empirical findings having their origins in the field of osteopathy and have yet to be scientifically validated. Chapman (Chapman 1936, Lines et al. 1990) discovered and described specific cutaneous and subcutaneous areas on the body that, when manipulated, can significantly improve organ function. Later, Goodheart, in trying to better understand these reflexes found that they could also improve specific muscle function. He noted that if he manipulated a Chapman reflex for a certain organ, it would change the surface temperature of the skin overlying the muscle associated to that organ. When temperature changes occurred, the underlying muscle would also strengthen (Goodheart 1965, Goodheart 1970). Since direct muscle–organ relationships have not been scientifically documented, the reflex mechanism causing these changes must be due to yet unknown cybernetic mechanisms in the body.

In part, the research above helped to determine the muscle–organ relationships that are now commonplace in AK. Once manual muscle testing has established an abnormal muscle response, the origin of the problem may be found using highly specialized, AK neurological assessment methods. More detailed discussions of the diagnostic procedures for identifying and resolving the origins of muscle dysfunction can be found in earlier AK texts by Walther (2000), Leaf (1996) and Garten (2012).

Within this book the anatomy, action and most important associations are represented along with a detailed description of precise testing procedures. After careful reading and upon gaining skill in the basic muscle testing procedures herein, the practitioner will be able to more specifically evaluate the causes of many structural problems. Even though the many therapeutic possibilities found in AK are not expressly discussed in this book, it should also be possible for the reader to potentially correct muscle dysfunction by cross-referencing them to one or more of the following:

- Related levels of motor innervation
- Organ associations and visceromatic reflexes
- Neurolymphatic reflexes for improving lymphatic drainage
- Neurovascular reflex points for greater vascular perfusion
- Acupuncture meridian associations
- Nutritional enhancement.

The art of manual muscle testing

For the most part, the tests used in PAK are similar to those found in the original text by Kendall. New variations to the original tests have improved their specificity and totally new muscle tests developed within AK are included as well.

Applied kinesiology primarily uses a patient initiated, isometric muscle test. It is extremely important that the patient be given enough time to arrive at a maximum contraction power prior to increasing resistance. During the initial stage, the examiner applies equal resistance to that of the patient, maintaining an isometric contraction. Should examiner resistance exceed that of the patient, false muscle weakness findings may result.

The patient's full isometric power is usually reached well within one second of the start of the test. At this point, resistance by the examiner is slightly increased causing a few degrees of movement of the limb upon which the muscle is acting (eccentric contraction).

The point of maximum isometric resistance is the most critical during testing. One of two responses can be noted. Either the tested limb 'locks' in the test position or is perceived to begin to move and 'give way'. The duration of the test normally should not exceed one second. If the patient is able to 'fix' the limb in place, one of two possible muscle states is

indicated. One, the muscle has a normal facilitation (normoreaction); a sign that nothing is amiss. Two, the muscle is in an over-facilitated or hyperreactive state. The hyperreactive state cannot be distinguished from the normoreactive until other testing criteria are added (see below).

Should the limb move from the start position, the muscle is deemed to have 'given way' and a hyporeactive dysfunction is indicated.

The ability of the patient to hold the start position throughout the test is dependent upon the integrity of both afferent sensory and efferent motor systems, as well as that from central regulation.

Performing the manual muscle test: basic principles

The main idea of the muscle test is to attempt to isolate the action of a specific muscle so that synergism from other muscles is eliminated or at least reduced to a minimum. In order to achieve this, the limb or body part that is acted on by the muscle is put into a precise start position. As a rule, this will be a position that approximates the origin and insertion of the muscle to shorten it by about one-half, thus allowing it to have maximum effectiveness.

Once the extremity is correctly positioned, the examiner takes a contact on the limb or body part as distally as necessary so that resistance is optimized without over-powering the muscle. Avoiding contacts over sensitive areas, especially on bony projections, is essential in order to prevent evoking pain that could cause a false weakness response.

The patient must be given clear and precise push or pull instructions so that the resistance direction strictly follows the arc of motion that the contracting muscle will impart on the joint. This is especially important when a muscle is functionally weak, as many individuals will experience difficulty in moving the limb in the direction indicated. This is one of the main reasons for 'patient initiated' testing. By allowing the patient to begin the movement, the examiner will be able to note deviations from the correct resistance direction prior to applying any counter resistance. On rare occasions, incorrect movement is due to the patient being confused rather than because the muscle is truly inhibited. When in doubt, it is best to repeat the instructions and the test up to several times in order to ensure success.

Resistance ability changes, often dramatically, from one subject to another. Ensuring that the test remains isometric is not always easy. The examiner must quickly and dynamically respond to the rapidly increasing strength of the patient so that an equal 'isometric' resistance is maintained. The patient reaches maximum isometric contraction when no further increase in power is felt. At this point, and not before, examiner resistance is slightly increased (usually for less than one second) converting the isometric contraction to an eccentric one. In this changeover phase, a slight movement of the joint as the isolated muscle lengthens will be noted. When in the presence of normal muscle function, the joint will begin to move, yet the test position is maintained, indicating an ability to adapt to the increased demand. When muscle weakness is present, the limb will move away from the start position. The movement vector of the limb when weakness is noted should optimally follow the arc of motion that the tested muscle would have on the joint. This is an indication of correct directional resistance by the examiner. During the transition phase from isometric to eccentric resistance, a muscle that is normal will have an elastic, yet firm, engagement pattern known as 'locking'.

Sources of error and precautions

'Isolation' of the muscle by controlling the test vector and position

Careful attention must be given to the test vector and is specific for each muscle. The vector is defined as the arc described by the limb should it be moved solely by the contraction of the tested muscle.

Hand contact by the examiner must be precise such that the direction of limb movement is guided by the sense of touch. Hand contact is best applied over as large an area as possible, often with a flat hand and approximated fingers. An overly firm grasp will often cause patient confusion as to resistance direction and/or provoke the examiner into using too much pressure.

Due to complex synergism between muscles, joint angles and positioning are paramount for muscle testing precision. A 'fine tuning' of the starting position will optimize the correct muscle length and help in isolating the main agonist. For example, the deltoid muscle is best tested with the shoulder in 90° of abduction while the synergistic supraspinatus should be tested, with preferably less than 30° abduction.

Neither the patient nor the examiner should make any alterations in contacts or body position during the test or when repeatedly testing the same muscle. When muscle dysfunction is already apparent, unconscious changes in limb starting position in order to recruit synergists is frequently noted. Changes can be extremely subtle, sometimes almost imperceptible, but can lead to significant changes in resistance capacity. The examiner must be meticulous in detecting these changes with visual and palpatory cues. When it does happen, or if one suspects that it has happened, the test should be repeated.

Stabilization

The patient's body must always be in a stable position and the joint acted on by the muscle firmly fixed in place. Gravity and the weight of the patient on the treatment table or a firm chair with a strong back are good sources of stabilization. Otherwise, the examiner provides the sole support, or, in combination with the above. Even the arm of a chair may be used, in order to avoid unnecessary recruitment as well as to impart on the patient the feeling that they can safely relax as much as possible.

Timing

For stand-up comedians timing is the most important factor in getting a laugh. Likewise, without proper timing in muscle testing, any diagnostic conclusion will tend to be more a joke rather than a serious finding. Timing is the most important and the most difficult skill to acquire. Some students will already be possessed of a well-developed sense of timing, but most will not. It is best to regard ourselves as 'unpossessed' of this ability until proven otherwise.

Timing is also dependent upon the exact direction of push or pull. The patient must be precisely instructed as to the direction of muscle contraction. Although these points have been mentioned above, they are of extreme importance and to mention them again will serve to reinforce their significance:

1. During the first phase of contraction, the examiner exerts only enough counter resistance to maintain isometric contraction.
2. When the contraction is felt to be no longer increasing, additional pressure is applied.
3. The additional pressure is made quickly, yet in a fluid fashion, without any sudden movement. The timing or 'feel' as to when to increase this pressure is essential.
4. Examiner resistance is released almost immediately upon sensing the 'locking' of the muscle.
5. When locking does not occur and limb movement is noted, muscle weakness is indicated.

Failure to release the limb when muscle locking is felt will tend to cause an increased lengthening of the muscle to a point greater than is desired or needed. Excessive stretch may put undue forces into the eccentrically contracting muscle – even in muscles that are normoreactive. The entire procedure, from the onset of patient resistance until the end of the test (when the examiner releases pressure) should last about one second and no more than 2 seconds. Although time differences might be minor, they are important and the total elapsed time is dependent upon the muscle being examined and each patient's inherent ability.

Contact hand positioning and 'lever length'

Leverage forces by the examiner should be adapted to the resistance ability of the patient. These forces are modulated in several ways. When testing muscles where there is a long lever, one may shorten or add to the lever length as desired or needed. This reduces the possibility of 'overpowering' the patient and provides for a more controlled test. With strong muscles (as those at surrounding the foot), contact is made as distal as is possible in order to gain more leverage. When the examiner is petit and the patient large and strong, body positioning as well as leverage must be used optimally. The examiner should always attempt to use the body ergonomically. Body positioning of the examiner is critical for reducing gross body movements and for enhancing sensory input from the testing hand and arm.

It is always a good strategy that the forearm of the examiner be placed such that the resistance direction vector will be in line with it. The test becomes more ergonomic for the examiner and helps the patient to achieve the most precise direction of resistance.

Instruction precision and mental forecasting

Patient instructions must be impartial and without indication as to what should or might happen. Instructions should be encouraging in order to achieve the best possible contraction. All tests must be performed without any expectation as to outcome (mental forecasting). In other words, operational bias must be kept to a minimum. Unconsciously or consciously predicting the outcome will undoubtedly lead to 'pilot error' by the examiner and falsify the test findings. Subtle, almost unperceivable alterations are automatically introduced and the test will 'appear' to be valid when it is not. The operator is most often unaware that changes in timing and resistive force have been made and the test result negatively influenced.

Breathing patterns

Muscle resistance can be significantly changed by breathing patterns. For example, is well-known and accepted that a deep inspiration during weight lifting enables one to a greater lifting potential. When the breathing pattern changes during muscle testing, it is usually noted in those patients who have a restrictive fault in the craniosacral respiratory mechanism, such as an 'inspiration assist lesion' (see Ch. 10 in Garten 2012, Leaf 1996, Walther 2000). A sudden inspiration or a breath cessation during testing should be taken as a possible 'respiratory assist' by the patient.

The temporomandibular joint and masticatory muscles

Malocclusion is relatively common. Clenching the teeth, especially coupled with a malocclusion, may alter the muscle testing response and falsify any findings. Even minor imbalances in occlusion or derangements of the temporomandibular joint (TMJ) are enough to cause barrage of mechanical and neurologic stressors into the body that will have wide spread negative consequences. Patients should be informed not to bite down during the examination. Clenching is an unconscious reaction and even though a patient has been told not to do it, it may occur. The examiner should be ever vigilant in restricting this tendency. The diagnostic challenges and workup of the occlusion and TMJ must be performed in a very controlled manner.

Patient hand placement

Uncontrolled, random touching of the body with the hands during testing should be avoided as it can lead to undesirable and erratic changes in the muscle tests. Early on, when AK was still in its infancy, the patient was allowed to place the hands wherever it was most comfortable. Goodheart observed that

hand positioning could alter the outcome of the muscle test. From these early observations the act of 'touching' a problem area is now considered to be a diagnostic provocation called therapy localization (TL).

Hand placement on the skin overlying a dysfunctional vertebra, organ reflex, and an active acupuncture, neurolymphatic or neurovascular point may cause a strong muscle to weaken or a functionally weak muscle to strengthen ('positive therapy localization').

TL is one of the 'holy trilogy' used in AK and without which AK would be a much less potent tool. Three basic diagnostic inputs, used in various combinations, are used to augment other, more classic diagnostic methods thus enabling the practitioner to obtain a more precise conclusion and therapeutic intervention. The precise manual muscle test occupies the top position of the triad and is the reference point from which all else is derived. The other two key factors are 'therapy localization' and 'challenge'. These phenomena transform the simple muscle test into a powerful clinical instrument that is without equal.

'Challenge' is the term used to describe the application of any sensory stimulus or provocation made that may affect the muscle testing response. Challenges are many and varied. They may be in the form of a simple manual directional pressure into an anatomical part or a complex array of chemical stimuli to the oral or olfactory senses. The diversity of challenge stimuli is immense. Some consider therapy localization to be a variation of challenge. 'Therapy localization' describes a situation whereby a patient's hand positioning on a body part will change previously tested muscle strength patterns. These specialized techniques are described in greater detail in Ch. 3 in Garten (2012), Leaf (1996) and Walther (2000).

Muscle fatigue and repetitive testing

Contractile strength and the ability to maintain a contraction are remarkably different between individuals. Thus, muscle fatigue must always be considered whenever attempting muscle testing. Muscle fatigue often develops when the examiner allows the patient's limb that to remain in the start position of the muscle test for too long a period of time. This is especially noted when testing muscles acting on a limb that is long and heavy as in the iliopsoas test. The novice examiner may not adequately support the leg of the patient prior to commencing the test and the weight of the limb will eventually exhaust the muscle. When the limb is easily maintained in the start position this is more rarely noted, but consideration with regard to a persons age and physical capacity should also be a factor.

Under normal circumstances, a muscle can be tested repeatedly at a rate of approximately once per second for at least 15 consecutive times without weakening. Upper extremity muscles may be tested at a more rapid pace and for more repetitions than than those of the lower extremities. In general, one is best served to apply the 15 times rule to all muscles. If the muscle tires sooner, it is most likely due to a disorder in aerobic or anaerobic muscle metabolism (see Ch. 10 in Garten 2012, Leaf 1996 and Walther 2000).

Summary of important criteria for manual muscle testing

Isolation of the main agonist (prime mover) by controlling the test position
Adequate stabilization
Avoiding recruitment
Patient initiated timing
Clear and precise patient instructions
Controlling adverse effects of malocclusion and the TMJ
Avoiding random hand placement
Control of testing hand contact
Inspiration and breath holding patterns
Observation of weakness through body language
Interpretation of muscle test outcomes: 'strong' vs. 'weak'

A muscle is perceived as 'strong' if it is able to resist the increase in dynamic pressure induced at the end of the isometric phase (keep the limb in the start position). A 'weak' muscle is described as being unable to 'lock into' or maintain the starting limb position at the point where increased force is induced.

The 'strong' muscle response must be clarified further because strong is not always normal. Any muscle able to maintain the test position is deemed to be 'strong' but may be either 'normoreactive' or abnormally 'hyperreactive'. In AK terms, 'normoreactive' indicates that the entire neuromuscular circuitry is functioning normally. Hyperreactive, on the other hand, is an abnormal muscle response indicating that there is some dysfunction due to a combination of chemical, emotional or electromagnetic stressors.

It is important to note, too, that there is a significant difference between hyperreactive and 'hypertonic' muscles. Therefore, it is imperative that they be clearly distinguished from one another. The hypertonic muscle is a separate entity both functionally and diagnostically and may test either 'strong' or 'weak'.

A muscle is deemed weak when the test position cannot be maintained. If the weakness can be subsequently changed by any therapeutic measure, the muscle is considered to be functionally weak. The functionally weak muscle is called 'hyporeactive'. Any muscle weakness that does not improve with any therapeutic input is most likely in a pathological state and referred to as such.

The following paragraphs delineate the criteria for their differentiation.

Normoreactive muscle

Diagnostic methods have been developed in order to insure that a muscle that tests strong is, in reality, normally strong rather than abnormally strong. It is important, therefore, to distinguish between normal and abnormal strong states. A muscle or muscle complex is described as 'normoreactive' when it can be functionally weakened (inhibited) by one of the methods described below. All of the many inhibition methods may be used to ensure that the muscle is normal, but in practice usually one or, at most two, are used due to practicality and time constraints.

Manual manipulation of spindle cells

The spindle cells in the area controlling the contraction of a muscle may be manually manipulated. Most often this is performed somewhere near the muscle belly. With large and long muscles like the quadriceps this area, ultimately depending upon the patient, might be a bit variable and a correct stimulus is ultimately dependent upon precision. At two points somewhere close to the centre of the muscle belly, a deep contact is made with the fingers of both hands. Pressure is applied along the muscle axis towards the belly from both points as if to compact the muscle tissue. When a muscle is normoreactive, it will weaken. It is hypothesized that the manoeuvre shortens the muscle spindles, temporarily down regulating them. The circuitry maintaining normal tonus is momentarily repressed, inhibiting the muscle contraction response to lenthening. The subsequent weakening of the muscle will last for only one contraction before returning to normal strength. This was one of the first procedures discovered by Goodheart and it was from this that the term 'normoreactive' muscle was coined.

Drainage (sedation) point stimulation

Most of the muscles have been associated with one of the acupuncture meridians. Goodheart found that changes in the energy pattern of a meridian can affect muscle function. When a digital or other form of stimulation is applied to the 'drainage point' of a meridian, the associated muscle will correspondingly weaken. The weakness is temporary and, like the spindle stimulation, it is considered a normal inhibition response. A simple manual percussion or a brief massaging is applied to the point just prior to muscle testing. Under normal circumstances, the sedation stimulus will cause an inhibition that can last anywhere from 10 s up to about 30 s.

Magnet effect

In the 1980s, it was found that a normoreactive muscle would weaken when a 3000 gauss magnet (= 3 $\text{Å} \sim 10^{-1}$ T) was placed over the belly of a muscle. The early magnets were flat and, being relatively large, were able to cover a large area of the muscle. Not all spindles are active at the same time, but the size of the magnet compensated for this by covering most of the muscle. Depending upon joint angulation and patient physiognomy, the active spindle cell area may vary. Smaller magnets must be accurately positioned for inhibition to occur.

The weaker, donut type ferrite magnet is in more common use today and, if incorrectly placed, will make the test unreliable.

It is most likely that inhibition is due to an alteration in local spindle cell signalling caused by the magnetic flux. The description of the polarity in AK follows the description of what is known as the 'technical' or 'medical' magnet as opposed to the 'geographical' terminology used in magnetic science.

In a small study, Angermaier describes how the 'medical' north pole of the magnet has an inhibiting effect that is consistent when blind testing is performed on the same patient and within the same parameters (Angermaier 2006).

Other methods for muscle inhibition

Other methods to test for normoreaction of a muscle have also been described in AK. One of the first used was that of 'backwards running of the meridian'. First described by Goodheart, it, and the spindle cell challenge, were the first methods discovered for verifying the normal muscle response. The examiner's hand is swept along the meridian starting from its highest and ending on its lowest point. Performed two or three times in rapid succession, a previously strong associated muscle is retested for strength.

Another, less known method, is to TL to the kidney 27 point on the same side of the body as the muscle being tested. This was investigated and proposed by Shafer (ICAK-USA Collected Papers 1982).

What Shafer found is quite different from the methods depicted above. The patient is asked to TL to K-27 on the same side of the muscle being tested. If it does NOT weaken, it is considered normal, whereas the opposite is true with the above mentioned tests. A weakening response would indicate a hyperreactive state. It should be noted that K-27 is used as a diagnostic point for functional neurological disorganization ('switching') as well. The hyperreactive muscle is usually caused by metabolic, emotional, electromagnetic or toxic stress. 'Switching' reflects this and the K-27 TL may be a form of 'super challenge' shifting a hyper to a hyporeaction.

Hyperreactive muscle

A hyperreactive muscle is defined as any muscle or muscle complex that cannot be inhibited by any of the measures delineated above for the normoreactive muscle; except that described by Shafer.

Early on Shafer coined the phrase 'over-facilitated' in an attempt to distinguish the abnormal muscle reaction from the otherwise used term 'hypertonic'. At about the same time, the word 'hyperreactive' was coined. 'Reactive', derived from the verb 'to react', is also used in reflexology and well describes this hyper response.

Thus, 'hypertonus' (Gerz 2000), 'over-facilitation' (Shafer seminar handouts) and 'conditionally hyperfacilitated' (Schmitt and Yanuck 1999) are all used in the same context. The difference between hypertonia and the concept of hyperreaction is dealt with in Garten (2012, Ch. 2.3). So that there is a clear and homogenous use of terminology in this text, the term 'hyperreactive' will be used exclusively throughout.

Finally, 'hyperreactive' must not be confused with the classic muscle dysfunction pattern called a 'reactive muscle'. First described by Goodheart, the reactive muscle is an abnormal spindle cell response in one muscle that causes an extended inhibition of its synergists or antagonists. Any muscle expressing prolonged inhibition was deemed 'reactive'. A reactive muscle, therefore, is not hyperreactive.

Hyporeactive muscle

Both the hyporeactive and weak muscle are defined as any muscle or muscle complex that cannot 'fixate' or 'lock' the body part in the start position against the examiner's resistance.

The hyporeactive muscle differs in that it may be capable of developing maximum isometric power (approaching strength 5 according to Janda (1994), see below). However, when the resistance changes from an isometric to an eccentric contraction, the muscle fails. The hyporeactive muscle cannot be evaluated with a force gauge device whereas the weak one can. For example, an athlete may appear to perform normally with respect to physical force ability, but in the presence of muscle hyporeactivity will be more prone to injury because of weak proprioceptive capacity. In severe cases, the hyporeactive muscle is unable to reach maximum isometric power (strengths 2 to 4 according to Janda) and will be similar to the weak muscle.

Most hyporeactive muscle responses will be immediately abolished when the appropriate therapy or suitable diagnostic challenge is applied. Following proper stimulus, the muscle will return to normal strength; although sometimes the change is only temporary. The muscle may return to normal or even become hyperreactive following therapeutic stimulus. According to Schmitt and Yanuck (1999), the muscle is then considered to be only functionally or 'conditionally' inhibited. This distinguishes it from the pathologically 'weak' muscle, whose inhibition cannot be immediately changed.

Dysreactive muscle

Any muscle that is abnormally functioning may be described as 'dysreactive'. Both hyper and hyporeactive muscle states are abnormal and are considered to be 'dysreactive'.

Weak muscle

A muscle, whose function cannot be improved by any therapeutic measure is deemed to be pathologically, not functionally weak.

Force interpretation according to a graduated scale

Applied kinesiology interprets predominantly the muscle reaction, not muscle strength. This appears to contradict Janda and Kendall who use a muscle strength grading system. The grading system was developed for neurological monitoring, where pathologies such as poliomyelitis and traumatic nerve damage were the main causes of muscle weakness.

Muscle testing as described by Janda and Kendall differs significantly from that in AK. The evaluation of a patient's resistance force can be very subjective and contrasts significantly with the functional testing of hyporeactive muscles found in AK. Thus, force gauges can be used with pathologically weak muscles, but not the hyporeactive.

Other questions arise as well. Kendall based strength parameters on what was reasoned to be the average adult. In order to accommodate childhood and early adolescence, arbitrary values were adopted. Thus anterior neck muscles of a 3-year-old child should have a value of about 30% that of the adult and a 5-year-old child about 50%. From there it rises gradually until the age of 10 or 12 where the standard adult value comes into effect (Kendall and Kendall 1983).

AK neuromuscular assessment allows for both functional disorders and pathologic states to be evaluated simultaneously. The professional athlete who trains daily may be assumed to have 'normal' strength values. But should the post-training increase in strength fall short of the expected, a functional disorder may be present. This is especially true if the athlete has been repeatedly injured and one may conclude that normal proprioceptive control is lacking. Only with the use of applied kinesiology testing methods do these types of muscle dysfunction become apparent.

Muscle strength grading was formally established and accepted by the British Medical Research Council (BMRC) in 1978 (see Table below) under the heading of motor function tests. These are very similar to the graduations found in Kendall and Kendall (1983) and Janda (1994).

The hyporeactive muscle according to AK testing may be compared to level 4– in the BMRC scoring, but often it may even be graded level 4+ or even 5. Levels 3 and 4 are also found in those experiencing difficulty standing on tiptoes or walking on the heals, i.e. have objective lack of force. It is recommended that an AK muscle evaluation (in terms of functional 'reaction') be made even when the graduated scaling method (for muscle force) is being used. In neurological deficits, regardless of pain (such as paresis of the arms, tetraparesis, cauda equina syndrome, intervertebral disc lesions and spinal compression), where surgical intervention is indicated but not concluded, AK muscle testing can help in arriving at a more precise conclusion as to whether conservative treatment might be favourable.

Motor function testing*

Grade	Definition
0	No muscle contraction evident
1	Muscle contraction barely visible with no movement noted
2	With gravity eliminated, slight movement noted of a part of the limb
3	Active movement of the limb against gravity
4–	Active movement against gravity and slight examiner resistance
4	Active movement possible against a resistance up to 75% of maximum
4+	Active movement against strong resistance, but weaker than the normal side
5	Normal movement against gravity and maximum resistance

*according to the British Medical Research Council (BMRC) of 1978 (mod. in accordance with Patten (1998))

Hypertonic muscle

In this book, the term hypertonicity is used in accordance with the medical literature and exclusively for muscles demonstrating an abnormally increased resistance to stretch and with an increased viscoelastic tone on palpation. The complex array of myofascial problems illustrates well the difference between hypertonicity and hyperreactive. Hypertonicity cannot be discerned using existing manual muscle testing methods.

Disorders of the pyramidal system causing spasticity and the extrapyramidal system causing rigidity are associated with hypertonicity. The causes for these lie in the central nervous system. Myofascial disorders, on the other hand, are peripheral causes of hypertonicity. Their origins may be due to overstrain and nociceptor reactions arriving from lesions in the locomotor apparatus. Naturally occurring pain mediators such as bradykinin may be released as a consequence of metabolic stressors and also cause hypertonicity.

Nociception causes muscle inhibition (Mense 2003, Mense 2004). The palpable, hypertonicity reaction due to nociception is commonly due to protective 'splinting'. Thus, the painful, palpably hypertonic muscle will be more often than not test hyporeactive.

Deep tendon reflex vs. manual muscle test

In theory, both the deep tendon reflex (DTR) and the muscle test assess the same neuromuscular circuits (see Ch. 12.2.3 in Garten 2012). The muscle test is far superior to the DTR as it detects even more subtle changes. Nevertheless, this does not exclude the value of the DTR and it should be an integral part of any examination. It is not uncommon to find an absent DTR, yet the muscle tests normal. Conversely, there are occasions where the muscle tests functionally weak and yet the DTR is intact. Perhaps this supports the concept that we are living, biological systems that do not always fit into a linear understanding.

This book is intended as a reference manual, not as a book focused on treatment options and modalities. Therefore only limited and specific therapeutic approaches are described for each muscle. They are deemed suitable for the normalization of hyporeactive muscles or for the relaxation of myofascially contracted (hypertonic) muscles. As a rule of thumb, most hyperreactive muscles will require a metabolic therapeutic approach for their resolution. More specific details of these methods are described in Garten (2012) and Garten and Weiss (2007).

Procedures for normalizing hyporeactive muscles

The seven factors of the viscerosomatic system

These consist of seven primary dysfunctional reflex relationships related to most muscles. The seven factors involved include motor function innervation, visceroparietal reflex relationship, neurovascular, anterior as well as posterior neurolymphatic reflex areas, nutritional components, acupuncture meridians and the associated organs.

1. Vertebral lesions

It is well known that vertebral dysfunction causes a nociceptive potential leading to an abnormal muscle response. This occurs for the most part through irritation of motor nerves that run through the intervertebral foramina (IVF) of a dysfunctional segment. Aberrant viscerosomatic reflexes due to irregularities found within organs, that in turn cause IVF and vertebral dysfunction, may also cause muscle inhibition. The complex inter-relationship between the viscera and the nervous system sets up a whole array of compensatory relationships that can be associated to the inhibited muscle.

In each case, all levels must, therefore, be tested and treated. Treatments often consist of high-velocity impulse manipulations and osteopathic techniques as well as special techniques of respiration-assisted mobilization used in applied kinesiology (Garten 2012, Leaf 1996, Walther 2000).

2. Neurolymphatic reflex points (NL)

The neurolymphatic reflex points are viscerosomatic reflex zones and were first described by Chapman (Chapman 1936 and described in Chaitow 1988).

Chapman reflexes are indurated (hardened) areas found in the viscerosomatic reflex zones related to an organ. They can vary from the size of bean up to several square centimetres. In more chronic cases, they often have a swollen appearance and oedematous stasis. Usually, the longer the disorder exists the greater the palpatory pain. Almost all of these reflexes zones or points are found on the upper body, the forearms and thighs. On the trunk they are located primarily in the anterior intercostal spaces and posteriorly along the vertebral column.

Chapman related these reflexes to the organs and Goodheart was the first to describe the therapeutic effect of the Chapman reflexes within the context of manual muscle testing (Goodheart 1965). He found that when manipulated as described by Chapman, they could eliminate muscle weakness. Goodheart had been already experimenting with muscle/organ inter-relationships and the Chapman reflexes seemed to support and confirm his hypothesis. Chapman stated that treatment of the reflex improved lymph drainage in and around the associated organ. This is what most likely inspired Goodheart to name them 'neurolymphatic reflexes'. In this manner the reflex zones described by Chapman became associated with specific muscle inhibition patterns.

Goodheart did not rely on muscle testing alone to understand the Chapman reflexes. He measured the surface temperature of the skin above a muscle related to one of the reflex zones. Upon manipulation of the reflex point, he noted time and again that the skin temperature would go down. He postulated that this was due to the lymphatic drainage effect of the manipulated reflex.

Treatment of a point or zone consists of relatively firm, circular motion massage, usually lasting 30 sec. Pain at the point should gradually subside throughout the therapeutic massage. Stimulation times of up to several minutes may be needed, but it is also important to avoid overstimulation. Overstimulation is not only unpleasant, but also detrimental to lymph flow.

3. Neurovascular reflex points

The so-called neurovascular reflex points were first described in the 1930s by Terrence Bennett. Bennett, like Chapman, found empirically that the points could influence the blood circulation in specific regions of the body and organs. Again, Goodheart used his understanding of muscle–organ relationships to assess the effect of these reflex points on muscles function. As with the Chapmen reflexes, he measured the skin temperature above the muscle related to a neurovascular reflex. Following appropriate stimulus to the point, he noted a significant increase in temperature as opposed to the decrease noted with the neurolymphatic point manipulation. He concluded that, indeed, this must be due to an increase in blood perfusion in the area. In this way he empirically established and identified the neurovascular reflex point for most muscles.

The treatment of neurovascular points consists of a gentle pull on the skin overlying the point. Contact is maintained until a slight pulsation can be felt and is usually noted after about 20–30 s. When points are bilateral, a synchronous pulsing should ideally be felt. For further details see Garten (2012), Leaf (1996) and Walther (2000).

4. Dural tension

In osteopathy, abnormal dural tension is the fundamental principle used to explain cranial and ilio-sacro-coccygeal imbalances as well as increased spinal torque. Muscle inhibition and dysfunction is always associated with abnormal dural tension; however, the relationship does not fit into any special pattern. Due to this it cannot be specifically systemized and does not make up a significant part of this book (for further details see Garten 2012, Leaf 1996 and Walther 2000).

5. Acupuncture meridian relationships

The acupuncture system was integrated into AK very early on by Goodheart and at a time when there was generally shown very little interest in acupuncture in the West (Goodheart 1966, Goodheart 1971). Meridian–muscle associations were not simply made to fit in accordance with the anatomically topographical relationships existing between the muscles and the meridians. Goodheart individually and painstakingly tested each muscle–meridian relationship. For example, the large intestine meridian is located on the arm, but the associated muscles are the tensor fasciae latae, the hamstrings and the quadratus lumborum. The muscle-meridian associations were established almost simultaneously with the muscle-organ associations (see above). Several of the meridians are not linked to specific organs and reflect a more a systemic rather than organ relationship. In Chinese medicine, the Sanjiao meridian (triple heater/warmer) does not have a specific organ associated. As well, not all organs were considered in Chinese medicine, as observed with the thyroid, thymus, adrenals, uterus, gonads and paranasal sinuses. In these cases classification was done using a meticulous, systematic series of tests. Goodheart empirically associated the Sanjiao meridian (triple heater) to the thyroid (teres minor) and the thymus (infraspinatus), whereas the adrenals, uterus, gonads where related to the circulation–sex (pericardium) meridian and the paranasal sinuses to stomach meridian.

The meridian relationships are described for each muscle under each chapter heading, but further explanation of this energetic relationship will not be dealt with in this text. For a more detailed discussion of this topic see Walther (2000) and Leaf (1996).

Fill point (tonification point, T):

Therapy localization is made on the tonification point for a meridian. If the TL normalizes a functional inhibition (weakness) of an associated muscle, the meridian is considered to be deficient in energy. Muscle inhibition, then, is often due to a void in meridian energy.

Drainage point (sedation point, S):

The drainage (sedation) point is described for those muscles, having a meridian association. Stimulation of the point, as described above, is important in determining the 'normoreactivity' of a muscle.

6. Muscle–organ relationships

These were established by Goodheart primarily in the time period from 1965–1967. A fortuitous combination from many sources lead to these conclusions. The Chapman and Bennett reflexes, along with his own personal observations melded together in helping him to formulate these very important connections. Empirically, he noted that patients with organ problems would evidence specific muscle weaknesses, which could be significantly improved as treatment for the organ or natural healing proved successful. For example, a toxic liver can lead to dysfunction of the pectoralis major sternalis and thyroid gland disorders can lead to dysfunction of the M. teres minor. Treatment protocols consist firstly of improving the metabolic function of the organ with orthomolecular, homoeopathic and/or allopathic products. Osteopathic type manipulation of the viscera may also be useful and necessary.

7. Nutrition

Goodheart found that appropriate nutrition could normalize neuromuscular function. Years of clinical application of these principles have reinforced these findings. There have been many empirical observations noting the important interrelationships found between muscles and optimum nutrient status of a patient. This has led to the definition of muscle–nutrient relationships in AK. Some of these relationships have been verified in studies (Carpenter et al. 1977, Leaf 1979).

Peripheral entrapments

Nerve entrapments lead to muscle weaknesses as well as to the development of hypertonicity patterns due to nociception. The weakness reaction may be easily muscle tested but the hypertonicity is generally determined by palpating or stretching the muscle. The peripheral compression sites affecting the muscles are cited in each chapter where entrapment syndromes are deemed important. Specific treatments must be appropriately designed to relieve the compression. With entrapment conditions the treatment protocol is not singular, but comprised of a multifactorial input. Often, it is necessary to relax hypertonic muscles, reduce irritation at the IVF and eliminate local oedema. For a more detailed discussion see Garten (2013) and other specific literature.

Proprioceptor disorders and nociceptor activation

Overactive inhibitory proprioceptors and nociceptors will lead to direct muscle inhibition patterns. These proprioceptors include:

- Golgi tendon organs
- Origin and insertion tendinosis
- Joint receptors of the peripheral joints.

Techniques such as deep friction and ultrasound are suitable for disorders of the muscle–tendon transition zones, while disorders of the peripheral joints are best treated using manipulation, mobilization and muscular balancing.

For details see Garten (2012).

Hypertonic muscles

The definition of hypertonicity is found above. The following are some notes and comments on the particular physical aspects relevant to the individual muscles and are important for the use of this book.

Myofascial syndrome

A myofascial syndrome is a condition of local muscular hypertonicity characterized by:

- Tense bundles of muscle fibres or 'taut bands' (Travell and Simons 1983)
- Trigger points characterized by a small focus of elevated irritability in a muscle or its fascia
- Referred pain patterns and other autonomic phenomena
- The pathomorphology of trigger points is characterized by actin-myosin-tethering. Tethering is a sign of lack of relaxation after contraction and in the long-term by degenerative changes in the muscle fibres themselves (Bergsmann and Bergsmann 1997).

Latent myofascial trigger point

Is clinically latent because there is no associated spontaneous pain and is only painful on palpation or by provocation by stretch and muscle contraction. The differential diagnostic limitations with regard to the active trigger point are therefore blurred.

Active myofascial trigger point

A muscle possessing an active trigger point will often have a specific pain or 'referred pain' pattern even at rest.

An active trigger point is always acutely sensitive and prevents full elongation of a muscle. It will weaken the muscle and with direct compression usually refer pain. When appropriately stimulated the trigger point produces a local twitching reaction of the muscle fibres that often leads to specific reactions in the autonomic phenomena of the vasomotor and sudomotor systems.

Chains of dysfunction

Muscle chains have their sensory and motor innervation originating predominantly by the same or by neighbouring roots. Trigger points found in a proximal muscle will frequently lead to satellite trigger points in more distal muscles of the same chain. The same leap-frogging can also occur in reverse. Frequently, trigger points have been found to correspond to the acupuncture points, thus making the muscle chain classifiable as a meridian of the acupuncture system. A muscle chain correlation is called a 'tendinomuscular meridian' (Garten 2013). The trigger point locations found in the muscle aid in determining its meridian

association. A 'distal point' lies on each affected muscle meridian. Abnormal activity of the distal point can affect the whole chain progressing above it. The distal points have been labeled on the diagrams in each chapter.

Referred pain

Referred pain either radiates from the site of lesion or is far removed from it. It may follow the cutaneous sensory dermatome and can also be attributed to a meridian.

Diagnosis and therapy

Myofascial syndromes often reveal themselves during the initial manual muscle testing. These muscles are frequently found to be painfully inhibited (hyporeactive). Most of the time they will also test 'weak in the clear'. Weak in the clear indicates that they will test weak without any additional provocation. It is probable that the muscle contraction during testing activates any trigger points that might be present. If the muscle does not weaken, hypertonicity may nevertheless exist. This can only be diagnosed with manual testing following a previously made diagnostic provocation. Goodheart found that if a hypertonic muscle was retested after stretching, it would become hyporeactive (Goodheart 1979).

Besides palpation, stretching of the muscle is the standard form of diagnosis for myofascial disorders. Along with this a comparison of the length of one side to the other is made as well as to weigh it against the empirical norm. The stretch position for each muscle are described and demonstrated in their relevant chapters.

Treatment options for hypertonicity are varied. Dry needling, spray and stretch and ischaemic compression may be used for trigger points. When muscle fascia is the problem, 'fascial flushing' (a muscle stripping massage according to Ida Rolf), or any of the osteopathic myofascial release methods as well as muscle energy techniques are applicable (Lewit 1992, Mitchell 1995–1999).

One of the most common techniques is post-isometric relaxation (PIR). The muscle is brought to its maximum stretch limit and held there under minimum contraction for 7–10 s. This is followed by gently bringing it to a new limit of length for another 10 s, but without active stretch. Breathing pattern may be used and are described in the specific sections for each muscle. For details see Lewit (1992), Mitchell 1995–1999 and Garten (2012).

Strain–counterstrain

Described by Jones (1981), it is not totally clear what this dysfunction might be. Most likely it is a form of muscular hypertonicity. On the other hand, it could possibly be just a particular form of therapy. The muscles having this dysfunction will demonstrate at least one, but usually more than one tender point. In contrast to trigger points, manual provocation of the tender points does not cause referred pain. The involved muscle is put into a position of maximum shortening for a period of 90–120 s. When held in the shortened position, palpatory pain over the tender point should be reduced by at least 70%. Additional components of rotation may be required. The shortened positions are not specifically indicated in this book, as they are easily derived from the muscle test position. The difference between the two is that the muscle test uses a mean shortening whereas the strain–counterstrain procedure has a near maximum shortening.

Spondylogenic reflex syndrome

The spondylogenic reflex syndrome was first described by Sutter and Dvorák (Sutter 1975, Dvorák and Dvorák 1991).

When segmental vertebral dysfunction or sacroiliac joint disorders are found, hypertonic reactions of a specific group of muscles will also develop. What is peculiar is that they are usually not directly linked to the irritated segment from which they are derived. For example, they are not associated to a muscle origin or insertion or its sensory-motor innervation. The afferent input for these reflex arcs originates from the nocireceptors found in the facet of the irritated joint. This relationship between muscle hypertension and the irritated segment were discovered by systematic investigation made by specific nociceptor provocation of individual intervertebral joints. Hypertonic saline solution or distilled water was injected into the joints in order to temporarily irritate the area.

Whenever a muscle is noted to be hypertonic upon palpation and for which local measures of muscular therapy are not effective, a spondylogenic reflex event must be considered. Where applicable, in each chapter, the spondylogenic reflex links to the muscles are given.

Basically there are logical sequences that cause dysfunction in muscular chains. AK follows the philosophy that muscular inhibition (hyporeactive muscles) is at the beginning of these chains. It is paramount that these be found and treated. Differential testing is then carried out to determine whether:

1. The antagonists to hyporeactive muscles have myofascial syndromes. These are characterized by a hypertonic shortening in the muscle due to a lack of inhibitory signalling from the hyporeactive functionally (weak) muscle. Normal agonist–antagonist inhibition is not present.

2. Synergists of hyporeactive muscles may show a type of strain reaction that resembles the strain–counterstrain pattern described above. This particularly applies to athletes whose injuries have been treated but where a full recovery has not taken place. For example, if an athlete begins too early to 'train up' the injured muscles, compensatory movement stereotypes and strains can result. The chain of events can occur in different sequences. Muscular hypertonicity may also be due to visceral irritation and result in excessive antagonist inhibition, usually affecting the synergists. There are, therefore, no fixed patterns, only certain guiding principles to the strain–counterstrain.

AK is inherently dependent upon a specific and accurate manual muscle test. Muscle testing ability is paramount to the ultimate success or failure in diagnosis. The decision was made to keep the theme herein restricted to muscle testing fundamentals rather than treating this vast subject in one enormous volume. On its face, muscle testing appears simple and this is what made it popular to the new age movement. Nothing could be more wrong. It is a delicate and finely tuned medical, diagnostic technique. George Goodheart used to say, 'It's simply complex and complexly simple'. In order to keep the complexities of muscle testing simple, this text allows the student to focus on learning the nuances of the muscle test. Experience shows that the neophyte student can become distracted into assuming that a precocious muscle testing ability is adequate and, filled with this false sense of bravado, attempt to make definitive diagnoses before this ability actually exists. It is for this reason that only a few adjunctive techniques, designed to enhance the understanding of muscles, muscle function and the muscle test, are discussed within these pages. More advanced techniques are to be found in other texts and publications on the subject and found in the bibliography that follows.

Overall layout of the muscle test pages

The muscle descriptions within this text are laid out in a unified fashion so that it is easier to look up and compare the individual aspects of each muscle. For ease of comprehension the main illustrations and muscle test description, whenever possible, have been placed on facing pages. Each muscle chapter has the same subheadings as those found below. Most of these are self-explanatory. Occasionally, a subheading will be absent and this indicates that it is not applicable to the muscle in question. The subheading order found below is the same for each chapter.

Origin, insertion and action

One might tend to quickly hop over these sections assuming that they are of little importance, but a clear awareness of muscle anatomy and function is extremely important. Without this specific understanding the limb will not be correctly positioned, the correct resistance vector will not be followed and false findings will result.

Signs of weakness

When muscle function is not in equilibrium the 'body language' of this is demonstrated in postural abnormalities. Signs of weakness have been added because postural analysis, as well as manual testing, is the best way to make the most specific muscle assessment.

Test

The test is initiated by the patient and this subheading explains the exact direction of resistance that is to be made by the examiner. The examiner must have a precise understanding of the appropriate resistance direction, be able to clearly explain it to the patient and be able to 'feel' if the appropriate movement is made. Take special note that the arrows on the illustrations always indicate the action or movement the patient must make, not the resistance direction of the examiner.

The seven factors of the viscerosomatic system

These are not found in every chapter. When included it indicates that dysfunction of the muscle in question is best evaluated by examining seven important factors as noted earlier.

To repeat, these are: motor innervation and visceroparietal vertebral levels, neurovascular and anterior and posterior neurolymphatic reflex areas, nutrition, the organs and acupuncture meridians.

Drainage point (sedation point, S)

Is important in AK for evaluating the normoreactivity of a muscle as opposed to hyperreactivity (over-facilitation). These points are illustrated and described for each muscle having a confirmed meridian relationship.

Fill point (tonification point, T)

Therapy localization (TL) may be made to the fill point linked to a weak (hyporeactive) muscle. When TL eliminates muscle weakness it is assumed that the meridian associated to the muscle is deficient in energy. Meridian balancing may rectify the problem. Should the weakness eventually return, it indicates that there remains an unstable electromagnetic aspect of the energy in the meridian system.

SR (spondylogenic reflexes)

Trigger points, myofascial gelosis, microlesions of muscles and other sensitive points are all painful on palpation. The spondylogenic reflex points or zones are painful as well and must be differentiated from the others. These zones are described in most muscle chapters.

Trigger points

The most common and frequently found trigger points for each muscle are illustrated and their relationships to nearby acupuncture points shown.

Effective distal points and tendinomuscular meridians

These are a group of peripheral acupuncture points that usually lie on a meridian having a segmental or topographical relationship to the specific muscle. The entire muscle chain collectively known as tendinomuscular meridians, will be influenced by the distal points. When stimulated, these points can have a beneficial re-equilibrating effect on muscles and muscle chains. The pain referral pattern corresponding to tendinomuscular meridians has also been included.

Strain–counterstrain

As described above, this is a muscle diagnosis and treatment technique originally developed in osteopathy and adapted into applied kinesiology (AK) by Goodheart. The neurologic theory behind the lesion's development and detailed evaluation procedures will not be described in this text. For this see Garten (2012) and Jones (1981).

Nevertheless, a general idea as to the evaluation of and test position for this important muscle lesion, may be derived, in part, from the individual muscle tests described in this text. Goodheart found that the lesion could be easily detected by using a specific, yet simple muscle testing procedure. The lesion is evaluated in almost the same manner as that described for the muscle test alone, but with one important difference. A muscle that has previously tested normal, but where the lesion is suspected, is put it into maximum shortening by the patient forcefully contracting it for a few seconds. A brief relaxation follows where the muscle is allowed to relax and the limb is then immediately returned to the rest position where it is retested in the normal fashion. Strain–counterstrain is confirmed should the muscle now test weak.

Stretch test

On the one hand, this test is relevant for diagnosis of muscle shortening and tightening and on the other hand, it can be useful in provoking referred pain originating from trigger points, thus making the diagnosis of myofascial and trigger-point-related problems easier. Limb positioning for the stretch test corresponds to the position used for the treatment of myofascial disorders, like the post isometric relaxation technique or when applying the spray and stretch therapy.

Post isometric relaxation (PIR)

Although PIR is not directly related to the muscle test, the decision to include this therapeutic modality within the text has proven popular. The method is appropriate for treating the hypertonic, shortened antagonist of a functionally inhibited agonist along with methods like fascial flush, dry needling, etc. Simple, yet effective, the relaxation procedure for each muscle, when applicable, is described. The arrows in the illustrations will always show the direction of contraction.

Anatomy

Origin: Over a broad area in the temporal fossa.

Insertion: At the apex of the coronoid process of the mandible with some fibres occasionally inserting on the disc and joint capsule.

Action

All fibres work together to elevate the mandible and close the jaw. Some protraction of the jaw is made by the anterior fibres and retraction by the posterior fibres.

Test

Is made indirectly with a strong (normoreactive) indicator muscle (NIM). Like with the masseter muscle examination, and unlike the pterygoid muscles, the patient can therapy localize (TL) directly over the muscle.

NIM indicator weakness with TL will be noted prior to applying any muscle challenges should there be active dysfunction at rest. A simple TL to the muscle will usually not lead to NIM weakness. Normally, the muscle must be actively tested.

As with all tests of the muscles of mastication, any premature contacts influencing the testing should be restricted by paper layers between the teeth.

The muscle is usually found to be hypertonic and passive elongation leads to the NIM weakness. It must be remembered that the muscle cannot be selectively isolated for stretch.

Myofascial syndrome

Stretch test (for all mandible elevators): The patient opens the mouth and attempts to fit three knuckles of the fingers between the incisors. The examiner assesses the elastic barrier of the joint and can lightly elongate the muscle further.

PIR: From the stretch position, the patient slowly contracts the muscle to close the jaw for 10 s during sustained inspiration. During the relaxation phase (in expiration) the examiner gently elongates the muscle by opening the jaw to bring it back and beyond the stretch position.

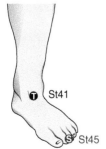

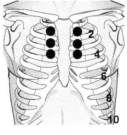

NL

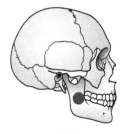

NV

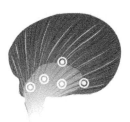

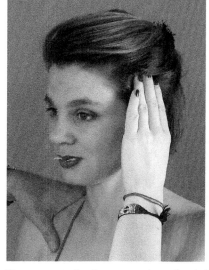

Motor function innervation:
Mandibular nerve (V)
Meridian: Stomach
Organ: Lymphatic system of the head
Nutrients: Vitamins C and E, beta carotene, selenium, iodine

Using a normal indicator muscle and with thin paper inserts between the teeth, TL is made over the temporalis during jaw closure

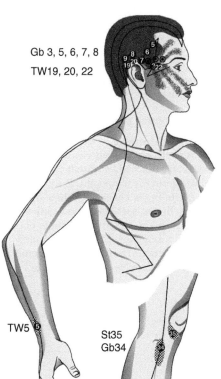

Gb 3, 5, 6, 7, 8

TW19, 20, 22

TW5

St35
Gb34

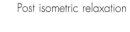

Post isometric relaxation

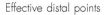

Effective distal points

Anatomy

Origin: Divided into two layers, superficial and deep; the superficial is larger. They insert one after another at the lower margin of the zygomatic arch of the zygomatic bone and at the zygomatic process of the maxilla. The superficial fibres are found more anterior on the zygoma and, the deeper fibres more posterior.

Course: The superficial fibres track from superior to inferior and somewhat posterior; the deep fibres run superior to inferior and slightly anterior.

Insertion: Angle of mandible, lateral side of the ramus of mandible and a few deep fibres insert on the coronoid process.

Action

Primarily closure and protrusion of the mandible, but the deep fibres also retract the mandible. The masseter muscle is more active when the biting force is applied to the molars as opposed to the incisors.

Test

There is no known direct test of the muscle. All testing is done indirectly with TL by the patient over the muscle. When the TL is positive, a NIM weakens during the test.

The accuracy of the procedure is dependent upon the elimination of confounding variables before starting the test. Prior to testing, it is best to place one to three layers of thin paper between the articular surfaces of the teeth. The procedure helps to reduce any false positive tests due to premature contacts. With the paper in place but still without TL, the patient is asked to bite down and the indicator muscle is tested. If weakness of the latter is noted, it is more likely due to gross dysfunction within the temporomandibular joint (TMJ) itself or other problems related to areas neighbouring the joint.

The paper sandwiched between the molars must not be too thick as it will tend to increase the vertical dimension (VD) of the TMJ. Increasing the VD with cotton rolls will elongate the muscle and possibly provide compensation for the shortening, which is the major common problem in the jaw elevators. It is, therefore, important to keep the thickness of the paper as thin as possible so as not to become a diagnostic challenge rather than a method to eliminate unwanted variables.

Evaluation is usually made with TL on the skin overlying the muscle during contraction or passive stretch, which will weaken a NIM in case of aberrant function of the masseter.

Myofascial syndrome

Stretch test (relates to all elevators of the mandible): The muscle cannot be selectively stretched because it cannot be isolated from the temporalis. It should be possible to fit the knuckles of three fingers between the incisors when the mouth is opened as wide as possible. If this is not possible, it is assumed that there is some jaw dysfunction. The examiner can gently elongate the muscles by attempting to

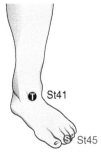

St41

St45

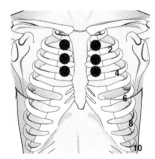

NL

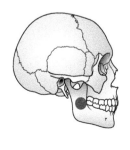

NV

manually open the jaw a bit more than the patient can manage. If a somewhat elastic endpoint is noted, the restriction is a soft tissue problem, most likely due to muscle contraction. A harder endpoint indicates that it is most likely due to articular derangement and caused by bony or discal resistance.

PIR: From the stretch position, the patient slowly closes the jaw to contract the muscle for 10 s during sustained inspiration. Following this, the examiner gently returns the jaw to the stretch position and slightly beyond during expiration, to elongate the muscle a bit more.

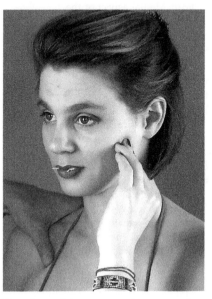

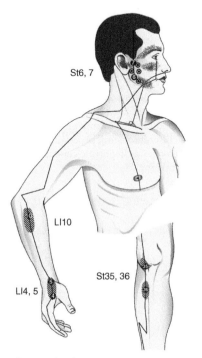

Motor function innervation:
Mandibular branch of the trigeminal nerve
Meridian: Stomach
Organ: Lymphatic system of the head
Nutrients: Vitamins C and E, beta carotene, selenium, iodine

TL and test of the masseter during jaw closure, using a normoreactive indicator muscle. Pre-contacts are neutralized by the strips of paper

St6, 7

LI10

St35, 36

LI4, 5

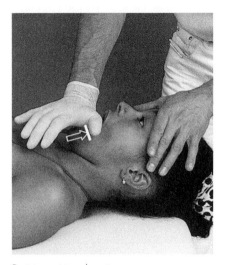

Post isometric relaxation

Effective distal points

Anatomy

Origin: Pterygoid fossa and maxillary tuberosity.
Course: Almost vertical with a slight posterior trend as it progresses inferiorly.
Insertion: Medial aspect of the mandibular angle.

Action

Closes and protrudes the jaw. With unilateral contraction, the jaw moves to the opposite side.

The fibres of the masseter muscle run on the outside of the ramus of mandible and those of the internal pterygoid on the inside making a sling-like attachment. A strong tendinous lamina joins the muscles at the junction of the lower, posterior margin of the ramus, thus forming a sling or 'masseter loop'. Working together, they are very strong elevators of the jaw. Even at rest there is an active tonus of the muscles. The TMJ is inherently instable which makes it similar, in some ways, to the glenohumeral joint. Like the supraspinatus muscle for the shoulder, a constant, low-grade tonus of these jaw muscles has been measured. The thought is that this is necessary to maintain a firm contact between the condyle, disc and the articular surface of the temporal bone. This is referred to as 'the loose packed position' (Farrar, in Schupp 1993).

Test

Like all the other jaw muscles, testing is indirect with the use of TL and an indicator muscle. The patient closes the jaw (firm bite) and therapy localizes the insertion of the muscle at the medial mandibular angle outside the mouth with the palmar side of the fingers. Hereby there is some limited access to the muscle as opposed to the lateral pterygoid which has none. Nevertheless, caution is advised when making diagnostic conclusions.

The possibility of premature contacts causing inhibition of a NIM weakness must be removed by the use of one to three layers of regular writing paper placed between the teeth as describe in the preceding chapters.

Again, it must be stressed that it is important to assess the effect of the paper layers prior to the actual muscle test. With the paper in place and without any TL, test NIM for weakening. The thickness of the paper is critical. Should the paper be too thick the change in vertical dimension of the joint may cause a diagnostic provocation and false positive findings for the muscle.

If there is a more pronounced malocclusion or possible TMJ compression problems, weakness will occur with the strips of paper in place and without TL. In these cases, passive stretch can be applied to the muscle. The positive response without TL is usually due to a hypertonic muscle and stretching will lead to a NIM weakness response. The muscle cannot be selectively stretched.

Test errors, precautions: Objective testing is limited at best. It is recommended that the examiner use a variety of different testing procedures in order to arrive at a diagnostic conclusion regarding this muscle.

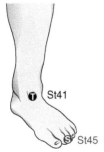

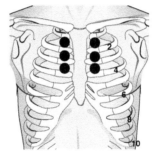

NL

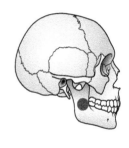

NV

Myofascial syndrome

Stretch test (for all mandible elevators): The patient should be able to fit three finger widths between the incisors when the mouth is wide open. As described earlier, the examiner can gently open the jaw further in order to elongate the muscle. If the muscle is shortened a relatively elastic endpoint is felt and when a bony or articular derangement is present, a harder endpoint is noted.

PIR: From the stretch position, the patient inspires and, while holding it for 10 s, slowly closes the jaw to contract the muscle. In the relaxation phase, the patient gradually breathes out while the examiner gently opens the jaw to elongate the muscle.

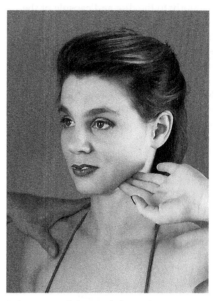

Indirect test of the medialis in the jaw closed position using TL and a NIM. Pre-contacts are neutralized by thin paper inserts between the teeth

Motor function innervation:
Mandibular nerve (V)
Meridian: Stomach
Organ: Lymphatic system of the head
Nutrients: Vitamins C and E, beta carotene, selenium, iodine

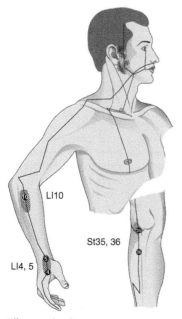

LI10

St35, 36

LI4, 5

Effective distal points

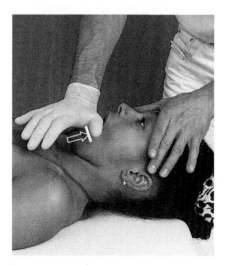

Post isometric relaxation

Anatomy

Origin: Superior head: Infratemporal surface of the greater wing of the sphenoid.

Inferior head: Pterygoid fossa and lateral surface of the lateral pterygoid process.

Course: Superior head: From the infratemporal surface downward and posteriorly to the disc and capsule of the TMJ.

Inferior head: Almost horizontally to the insertion.

Both heads follow a general path that angles approximately 45° from an anterior and medial origin, then posteriorly and laterally to the insertion.

Insertion: Superior head: Articular disc and joint capsule.

Inferior head: On the neck of mandible just below the condyle.

Action

Superior head: More active during jaw closure and controls the 'return speed' of the articular disc and the condyle as well, if there is an insertion on the neck of the mandible (Schupp 1993, Siebert 1995). As the jaw closes, the contractile tone of the muscle increases significantly.

Inferior head: With unilateral contraction, the mandible will move to the opposite side (laterotrusion). During bilateral contraction, protrusion and jaw opening takes place. The muscle has no residual activity when the jaw is closed.

Test

Is an indirect test made by the use of a NIM and TL made as close to the muscle being evaluated as is possible. TL is made with the patient's finger inside the mouth in the cul de sac found between the maxillary tubercle and the coronoid process.

Alternative: TL is made externally on the TMJ during protrusion or laterotrusion. A positive TL may be noted on either side in any position due to the fact that the joints work together.

TL should not be positive over the TMJ when in a relaxed, closed position. If TL with the jaw in a closed, resting position causes an indicator muscle to weaken, and this weakness is eliminated when the patient moves the jaw laterally to the right, it might be due to a hypertonicity of the right lateral pterygoid. The hypertonic muscle tends to keep the jaw more to the left and by moving the jaw to the right, the positive TL is eliminated because the abnormal muscle activity is dampened.

When TL remains positive, some other component or pathology might be present.

Functional evaluation

Simultaneous TL is made to both TMJ's and the patient is instructed to protrude the jaw. If a NIM weakens, laterotrusion of the jaw is used to identify the side of involvement. For example, if laterotrusion to the right weakens a NIM, it can be indicative of left lateral pterygoid hypertonus. Right laterotrusion contracts the muscle, activating any myofascial dysfunction and causes a NIM to weaken. As well, the simultaneous stretching of the right lateral pterygoid muscle may also cause the NIM to weaken. Both sides should be carefully examined and treated even though only one side tests positive.

Myofascial syndrome

Stretch test: Not possible.

PIR: With the patient supine the examiner takes a light contact to the anterior mandible below the lower lip. The patient, while sustaining an inspiration for about 10 s, is instructed to gently push the jaw forward against light resistance by the examiner. In the relaxation phase the patient breathes out while allowing the jaw to loosely drop back to a relaxed position.

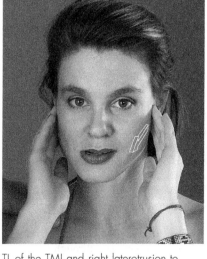

Motor function innervation:
Mandibular nerve (V)
Meridian: Stomach
Organ: Lymphatic system of the head
Nutrients: Vitamins C and E, beta carotene, selenium, iodine

TL of the TMJ and right laterotrusion to activate the left lateral pterygoid. A normoreactive indicator is tested for weakening

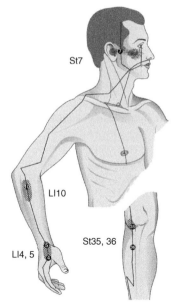

St7

LI10

LI4, 5

St35, 36

Effective distal points

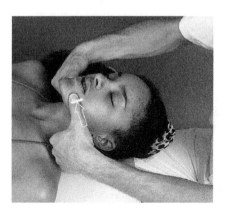

Post isometric relaxation

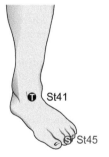

St41

St45

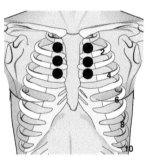

NL

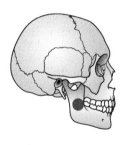

NV

Anatomy

Origin: Posterior belly: Medial to the mastoid process on the nuchal line and from a deep, 'digastric' groove between the mastoid and styloid processes of the temporal bone.

Anterior belly: From the digastric fossa at the medial, lower border of the mandible.

Course: Posterior belly: From posterior to anterior and inferior.

Anterior belly: From anterior to posterior and superior.

Insertion: Both bellies insert into a common, central tendon by a fascial loop formed as they pass through the stylohyoideus muscle connecting to the body of the hyoid bone.

Action

Opens the jaw and lifts the hyoid bone. When the hyoid bone is fixed, it aids in depressing the mandible. The digastric muscle is interesting in that while it is considered a single muscle, the bellies have separate embryologic origins. The anterior belly is innervated by the 3rd division of the trigeminal nerve, while the posterior belly is innervated by the digastric branch of the facial nerve. Paresis of one of the two nerves will still allow some elevation of the hyoid by the other.

Test

As with the other muscles of mastication, this test must be performed indirectly using TL and a NIM. The jaw is held open and the patient therapy localizes to the muscle. A NIM will weaken with muscle dysfunction.

A stretching challenge to the muscle is often the most practical here. Using a sustained challenge, the hyoid bone is pulled down and laterally while the patient therapy localizes the muscle. A NIM will weaken when myofascial disorders are present.

Myofascial syndrome

Stretch test: Is best made by using the stretching challenge as described above.

PIR: Stabilize the patient's chin below with one hand and with the other hand pulls the hyoid bone down to the point where the positive challenge was noted. The patient holds a sustained inspiration for about 10 s while slowly and gently opening the mouth. During the relaxation phase, and without resistance by the examiner, the patient slowly exhales while returning the jaw to the closed position.

Stylohyoid muscle

Anatomy

Origin: Styloid process of the temporal bone.

Insertion: To the body of the hyoid at the border of the greater horn.

Action

Lifts the hyoid and pulls it posteriorly.

Test

Some perform this test without TL and others believe that TL is needed. Here it will be described without TL. The hyoid bone is pulled forward and down, then released. A NIM will weaken if a myofascial problem is present in the muscle.

The posterior belly of the digastric muscle is very similar to the stylohyoid muscle with respect to its course and action on the hyoid. The difference is found during contraction. The combined actions of both bellies of the digastric muscle tend to pull the hyoid superior (and possibly somewhat anterior), whereas the stylohyoid pulls the hyoid in a more posterior and superior direction. An attempt should be made by the examiner to pull it anterior and laterally instead of straight down.

All reflex points for the stylohyoid are the same as those for the digastric muscle.

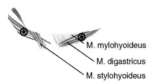

M. mylohyoideus
M. digastricus
M. stylohyoideus

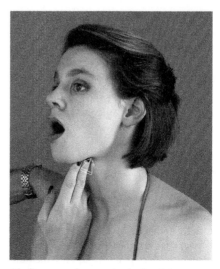

Motor function innervation:
Digastric muscle: Mandibular division of the trigeminal – anterior belly, facial nerve – posterior belly
Stylohyoid muscle: Facial nerve
Mylohyoid muscle: Mandibular branch (V)
Geniohyoid muscle: C1 via hypoglossal nerve
Organs: Head – lymphatic system
Nutrients: Vitamins C and E, beta carotene, selenium, iodine

Challenge to the anterior belly of the digastricus on the left. A NIM is tested for strength

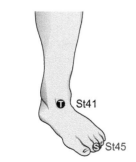

St41
St45

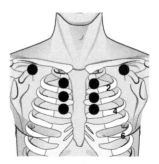

NL anterior

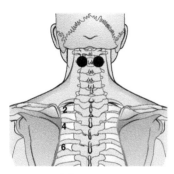

NL posterior

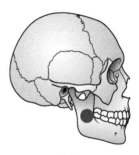

NV

Mylohyoid muscle

Anatomy

Origin: From the mylohyoid line of the mandible.

Course: The flattest muscle in the floor of the mouth, lying directly below the digastric muscle, converging medially and posteriorly.

Insertion: In the middle of the hyoid body.

Action

Lifts the diaphragm-like floor of the mouth, opens the jaw and lifts the hyoid bone. When contracted bilaterally, it provides a firm platform upon which the tongue can push.

Test

The patient presses the tongue against the hard palate while TL is made to the floor of the mouth from the inside or from the outside, submandibularly. A previously NIM is tested for weakness. Dysfunction of the mylohyoid muscle will cause a dysreaction (weaken) of the NIM. The TL may also be positive in the resting position of the jaw. When this is the case, a diagnostic differentiation must be made between muscle dysfunction and a possible lymph drainage disorder of the jaw. A lymphatic nosode challenge (Garten 2004, Garten and Weiss 2007) will help in distinguishing between the two very different aetiologies.

All reflex points for the mylohyoid are the same as those for the digastric muscle.

PIR: With the jaw open, the patient holds a sustained inspiration for 10 s while pressing the tongue against the hard palate. During the relaxation phase, the tongue is brought down to its resting position while the patient slowly breathes out.

Geniohyoid muscle

Anatomy

Origin: Behind the posterior tip of the chin.

Course: Lies one layer deep to the mylohyoid muscle.

Insertion: On the hyoid bone.

Action

Opens the jaw and lifts the hyoid bone.

Test

A specific test is impossible as the muscle is a direct synergist of the digastric and mylohyoid muscles.

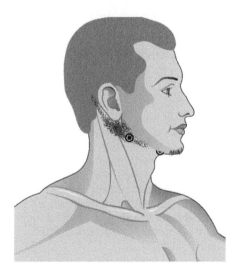

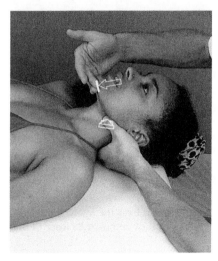

Trigger point of and referred pain from the digastric muscle

Post isometric relaxation

Sternohyoid muscle

Anatomy

Origin: Posterior surface of the manubrium of sternum and sternal end of the clavicle.
Insertion: Inferior margin of the body of the hyoid bone.

Action

In a combined action with the three muscles below, it fixes the hyoid inferiorly and depresses it by bringing it closer to the sternum.

Sternothyroid muscle

Anatomy

Origin: Manubrium of sternum and cartilage of the 1st rib.
Insertion: Oblique line of the thyroid cartilage.

Action

Fixes the thyroid cartilage inferiorly and depresses it by bringing it closer to the sternum.

Thyrohyoid muscle

Anatomy

Origin: Oblique line of the thyroid cartilage.
Insertion: At the hyoid bone at the border with the greater horn of the hyoid bone.

Action

Approximates the hyoid bone and thyroid cartilage.

Omohyoid muscle

Anatomy

Origin: At the upper margin of the scapula.
Course: Both bellies are linked with a tendon found just below the sternocleido-mastoid muscle. From the origin, it slants slightly forward and upward passing underneath the clavicle, diagonally over the front of the neck and superior to the brachial plexus to its tendon beneath the sternocleidomastoid muscle. From this point it progresses almost vertically to its insertion on the hyoid.
Insertion: Lateral part of the major horn of the hyoid.

Action

Lowers the hyoid bone and pulls it backwards, dorsally.

Myofascial syndrome

A hypertonic omohyoid muscle in association with trigger points can cause brachialgia due to its course near the brachial plexus and may mimic a compression syndrome at the thoracic outlet (see also scalene muscles).

Test of the infrahyoidal muscles

The applied kinesiology hyoid challenge is probably the best diagnostic option available. The hyoid is held between the examiner's thumb and index finger and the lateral borders are displaced using a sustained or non-sustained challenge. The various challenge directions (upwards, lateral and medial) will provoke different fibres. A NIM will weaken when myofascial disorders are present.
TL over the different muscles will aid in determining the involved muscle.

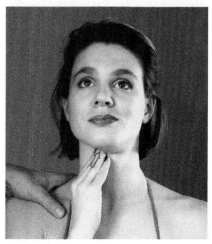

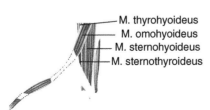

— M. thyrohyoideus
— M. omohyoideus
— M. sternohyoideus
—M. sternothyroideus

Challenge of the right omohyoid muscle. A NIM is tested

Motor function innervation:
M. thyrohyoideus: C1, 2 via hypoglossal nerve
M. omohyoideus: C1, 2 via hypoglossal nerve
M. sternohyoideus: C1, 2 via hypoglossal nerve
M. sternothyroideus: C1, 2 via hypoglossal nerve
Organs: Lymphatic system of the head
Nutrients: Vitamins C and E, beta carotene, selenium, iodine

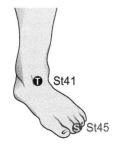

St41

St45

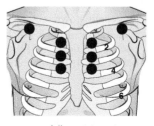

NL anterior

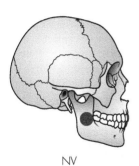

NV

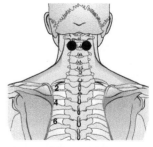

NL posterior

M. obliquus internus abdominis

Anatomy

Origin: Lumbar aponeurosis, iliac crest and lateral half of the inguinal ligament.

Course: Diagonally upward and anterior. The posterior fibres arch more medially and the anterior fibres progress in an increasingly horizontal fashion. Lies between the obliquus abdominis externus and transversus muscles.

Insertion: The posterior fibres insert on the three to four lower ribs and the more anterior fibres radiate into the rectal sheath of the rectus abdominus. The most inferior fibres of the anterior part pass through the inguinal canal together with the spermatic cord to become the cremaster muscle.

M. obliquus externus abdominis

Anatomy

Origin: At the lateral surface of the lower eight ribs.

Course: Diagonally down and medially.

Insertion: The superior fibres radiate into the rectal sheath and the lower fibres insert at the iliac crest and the inguinal ligament.

Action

With bilateral contraction, the symphysis and the thorax converge, the abdominal wall becomes more rigid and the intestines are held in place.

When a coupled simultaneous contraction of the internal oblique on one side and the external oblique on the opposite side is made, the vertebral column and trunk are rotated and laterally inclined.

Signs of weakness: According to Mayr (Rauch 1994), if the lower fibres are weak a 'paunch' develops. Bilateral weakness will produce an anterior tilt of the whole pelvis and a one-sided weakness will cause an anterior ilium displacement on the involved side. A bulging of the lateral abdomen when sitting up may also be noted.

Test

Anterior fibres

The obliquus externus and the contralateral obliquus internus abdominis are tested at the same time for all of the tests. Each muscle is dependent upon the other for its action and it is impossible to isolate them from one another.

Position: The trunk is flexed about 75° and rotated approximately 45° to one side or the other. With the trunk rotated to the left where the right shoulder is rotated forward, the right externus and the left internus muscles are tested.

When the trunk is flexed to 90°, the inferior fibres are tested. It is important to note here, that the increased flexion of 15° will significantly change the resistance direction by the examiner. Resistance must begin by the examiner pushing slightly cranially with the contact hand and always following the arc of the trunk as it descends toward the table.

Stabilization: The patient's legs should be firmly fixed on the table in an extended or in a slightly bent position.

Test contact: The patient's arms are crossed so that the hands are in contact with the opposite shoulders. The examiner takes a broad contact on the arms and elbows as they cross over the centre of the chest. The contact is made as distally as is comfortably possible.

The externus can be somewhat better isolated and differentiated from the internus, if the contact is moved to the anteriorly rotated shoulder instead of centrally at the crossed elbows. The pelvis and legs must be well stabilized on the table surface.

The internal oblique is emphasized more when the resistance contact is moved to the side of the posteriorly rotated shoulder.

Patient: While exhaling, flexes the trunk anteriorly by bending forward towards the feet as if to finish a sit-up.

Examiner: Resists further flexion, by pressing the trunk back.

Note: An alternative test can be made that is similar to the recommended training method for the abdominal muscles. With

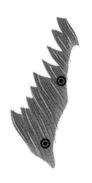

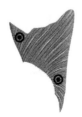

M. obliquus externus abdominis   M. obliquus internus abdominis

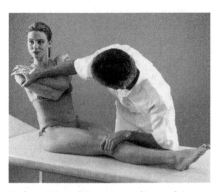

Preferred test of the anterior fibres of the
external oblique muscles on the right

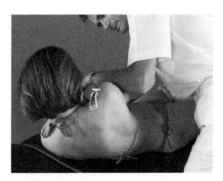

Alternative test for the oblique abdominal
muscles

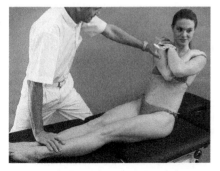

Preferred test of the anterior fibres of the
internal oblique muscles on the right

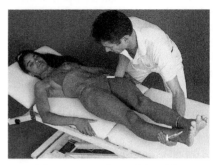

Test of the posterior fibres of the oblique
abdominal muscles on the right. The legs are
lifted about 15 cm from the table

the arms crossed over the chest and the legs firmly fixed to the table surface, the supine patient contracts the abdominal muscles without flexing at the hip, so that the upper trunk is lifted from the table. With the trunk elevated, it is then rotated fully to the side opposite the test. The examiner, contacting the anterior aspect of the elevated shoulder, tries to push it backwards towards the table. Stabilization and fixation of the legs and hips is much more difficult with this test due to the distance from the point of fixation and test contact. With long patients and short examiners, stabilization may be only possible with the help of another person.

Test errors, precautions: If the examiner selects a resistance point that is too far down on the trunk, the lever is severely shortened and the muscles will test falsely strong. A resistance vector made in a slightly more cranial direction may help to avoid too much recruitment of the synergistic psoas muscles. Expiration increases the relative strength of the muscle and may help weaker patients to make a more forceful contraction. The more the lumbar spine is flexed, the more the psoas muscle will be recruited.

Posterior divisions of the Mm. obliqui abdominis

Position: With the patient in a supine position, the legs are lifted about 15 cm from the table and the trunk laterally flexed by 10° to the side being tested. The examiner is positioned on the side of the body opposite to the muscles being tested.

Stabilization: At the lateral aspect of the hip that is closest to the examiner and opposite the side being tested.

Contact: The arm is placed underneath both legs as close to the ankles as is physically possible for the examiner. With the legs supported by the arm, the examiner curls the fingers up and wraps them around the opposite, more distant leg so that both may be pulled together. The testing arm under the legs helps to keep them elevated from the table during the test.

Patient: Keeping the legs slightly elevated, draws the legs to the side away from the examiner.

Examiner: Stands or sits on the opposite side of the test in the same fashion as with the quadratus lumborum test. Resists by simultaneously pulling the legs and pushing on the pelvis attempting to straighten the body.

Watch for pronounced synergism of the quadratus lumborum. The quadratus lumborum is tested with the legs flat on the table and the only difference in the test is the slight elevation of the legs. Body rotation, seen by rolling the trunk to the tested side, should also be avoided.

Myofascial syndrome

Stretch test: The examiner places a knee on the table, next to the seated patient's pelvis, opposite the side to be stretched. The arm on the side to be tested is flexed at the elbow and the elbow lifted above the head. The elbow is grasped and used as a lever to bend the trunk laterally over the examiner's thigh to stretch the abdominals. The patient sustains an inspiration to relax the abdominal muscles, while the examiner holds the trunk down. All muscles of the lateral abdominal and chest wall will be stretched. The posterior or anterior divisions can be stretched more precisely by imparting a flexion or extension component to the trunk during the sidebending.

PIR: From the stretch position, contraction can be elicited by instructing the patient to look up to the side of the stretch while simultaneously exhaling. The abdominal muscles automatically contract when breathing out. In the relaxation phase the patient inhales and looks down and to the side opposite the stretch, while the examiner gently returns the trunk and arm to the stretched position. The elbow is again used as a lever to laterally bend the body over the knee.

Frequently found associated disorders

Chronic instability of the pelvis with low back pain due to anterior displacement of the ilium and hyperlordosis of the lumbar spine. Digestive disorders may influence the muscle as well.

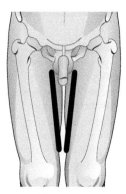

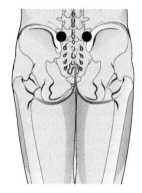

NL anterior   NL posterior

Trigger points of the oblique muscles and
referred pain pattern

Motor function innervation: T7–T12
Viscerosomatic segment: T6–T7
Rib pump: Intercostal space, costotransverse
joint 1, 2, 7 and 10
Meridian: Small intestine
Organ: Small intestine
Nutrients: Vitamin E, coenzyme Q10,
probiotics (lactobacillus, etc.)

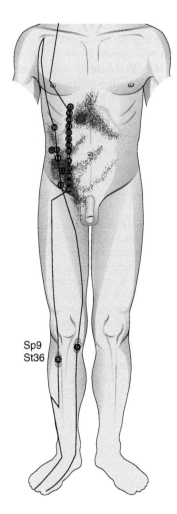

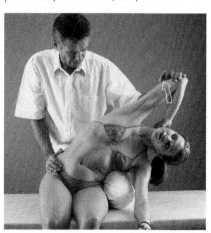

Sp9
St36

Post isometric relaxation from the stretch
position with expiration, upward gaze and
contraction

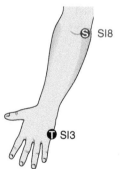

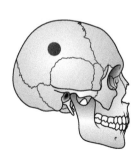

NV

Anatomy

Origin: Superior margin of the pubic bone between the pubic tubercle and the symphysis.

Course: Widens as it progresses vertically upwards. In the middle, it is divided by three interdigitating tendons.

Insertion: On the chondral part of the 5th to 7th ribs and the xiphoid process.

Action

Approximates the sternum and the symphysis pubis, stabilizing the pelvis anteriorly from posterior rotation. Together with the obliquus abdominis it stabilizes the abdominal viscera. Relaxes on inspiration and contracts with forced expiration.

Signs of weakness: Anterior tilting of the pelvis. With pronounced weakness of the upper segments there is protrusion of the upper abdomen as seen in a pot-belly type meteorism according to Mayr (Rauch 1994). With weakness of the lower segments, a protrusion of the lower abdomen is noted as a paunch or seed-sower posture according to Mayr.

Test

Position: The patient sits upright with the knees straight or bent at about 45°. An attempt to maintain a normal lordosis of the lumbar spine should be made. The patient crosses the arms in front of the chest and turns the trunk only slightly, about 10°, to the opposite side of the muscle to be tested.

Test contact: To the patient's crossed arms and slightly more toward the side of truncal anteriority.

Stabilization: Over both legs as distal as is physically possible depending upon examiner body proportions.

Patient: Breathes out and flexes the trunk down towards the pelvis and thighs.

Examiner: Resists the flexion. This is a more difficult test than would be initially assumed. The pressure vector must follow the arc that the trunk makes when flexing in this position. Pressure is best applied at first from a more inferior to superior direction and then, when weakness is noted, the angle becomes more anterior to posterior.

With greater flexion of the trunk (80–110°) the lower segments are tested and with less flexion (45–80°) the upper segments become more active. If both divisions are tested simultaneously, the patient's trunk is placed in a neutral position with no imparted rotation.

Alternative test: Even with the knees bent the psoas is an extremely strong synergist in the abdominal muscle test. As opposed to the above test, the supine patient is asked to cross the arms over the chest and only lift the chest from the table, as if to do a 'stomach crunch' rather than a sit-up. The examiner makes contact on the crossed arms trying to press the patient's upper body away from the symphysis and towards to the table.

Test errors, precautions: If the examiner uses a contact that is too far down the body, the lever resistance forces will be severely shortened and false negative tests will likely ensue. It is extremely important to follow the proper vector, reminding oneself that the abdominals move the xyphoid towards the symphysis. Expiration increases the relative strength of the muscle. As the lumbar spine is progressively bent forward, the psoas muscle is increasingly recruited.

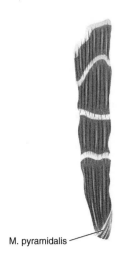

M. pyramidalis

Motor function innervation: T5–T12
Viscerosomatic segment: T6–T7
Rib pump: Intercostal space, costotransverse joint 3, 5 and 10
Meridian: Small intestine
Organ: Small intestine
Nutrients: Vitamin E, coenzyme Q10, probiotics (lactobacillus, etc.)
SRS: Symphysis lesions (inferior sections)

Rectus abdominis and pyramidalis muscles

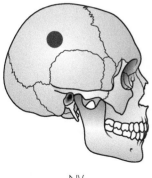

NV

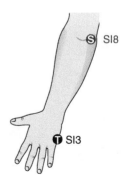

S SI8

T SI3

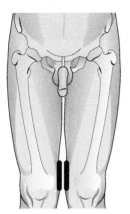

NL anterior

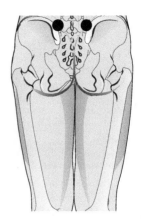

NL posterior

Myofascial syndrome

Stretch test: Is made by imparting a hyperlordosis in the lumbar spine. Placing a large cushion underneath the spine in the supine patient, or, when in the prone position, the trunk is pushed into extension. Nevertheless, the test is not very significant as many factors, including lumbar osteoarthritis, may influence extension.

PIR: Not applicable.

Cause for compression: The anterior branch of the spinal nerve can be irritated by local trauma as it passes through the rectus abdominis. Eventually this leads to parietal or even visceral pain in the area of the involved segment.

Frequently found associated disorders

According to Goodheart (1979), cranial bone restrictions of the sagittal suture, usually of a compressive nature, have been associated with bilateral rectus adominis inhibition (Walther 1983, Walther 2000).

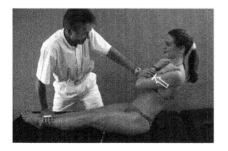

Right rectus abdominis test (superior fibres or divisions)

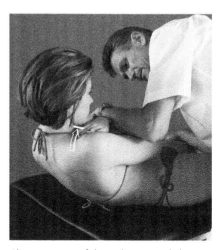

Alternative test of the right rectus abdominis

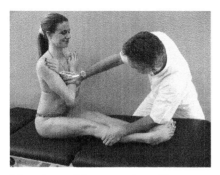

Bilateral test of the more inferior fibres or divisions, including pyramidalis. The extended arm is a more ergonomic position for the examiner

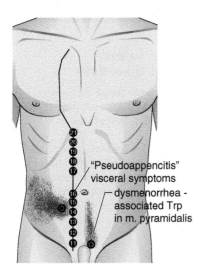

Trigger points and referred pain pattern for the rectus abdominis

"Pseudoappencitis"
visceral symptoms

dysmenorrhea -
associated Trp
in m. pyramidalis

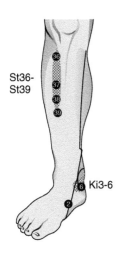

St36-
St39

Ki3-6

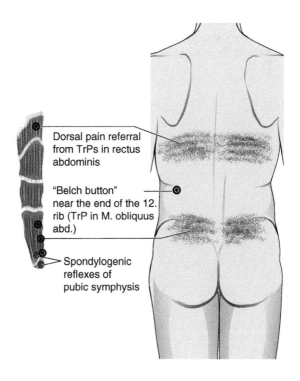

Dorsal pain referral
from TrPs in rectus
abdominis

"Belch button"
near the end of the 12.
rib (TrP in M. obliquus
abd.)

Spondylogenic
reflexes of
pubic symphysis

Anatomy

Origin: On the flexor retinaculum, tendon of the flexor carpi ulnaris, pisohamate ligament, and the pisiform bone.

Course: Progresses in a straight line from the origin to its insertion and is the muscle of the ball of the little finger that is closest to the ulna.

Insertion: Ulnar side of the base of the proximal phalanx of the little finger and at the dorsal aponeurosis.

Action

Abducts and helps with opposition of the little finger, as well as bending of the proximal phalanx.

Test

Position: Abduction of the little finger.

Stabilization: Fixation of the patient's hand from rotation and other contorsional movements.

Test contact: The examiner places the testing finger on the ulnar side of the middle phalanx of the little finger.

Patient: Abducts the little finger.

Examiner: Using great sensitivity, pushes the little finger in adduction.

Frequently found associated disorders

Compression weakness: Pisiform hamate and sulcus ulnaris syndromes or any other proximal compression of the ulnar nerve.

The abductor digiti minimi is often more accurate and is a more definitive diagnostic indicator for compression syndromes of the ulnar nerve than the opponens digiti minimi. It is also good for the evaluation of C8 root compression.

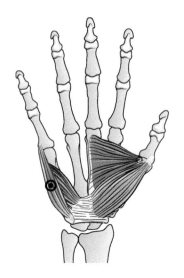

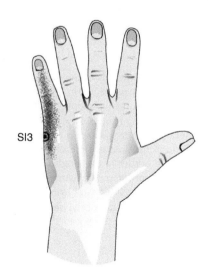

SI3

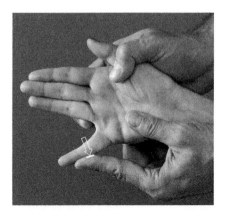

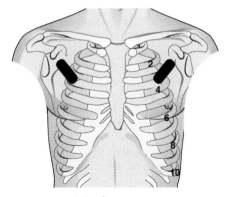

NL reflex anterior

Motor function innervation: Ulnar nerve, C(7), C8, T1

Anatomy

Origin: Medial process of the calcaneal tuberosity, flexor retinaculum, plantar aponeurosis and medial plantar septum.

Course: Running from posterior to anterior on the internal aspect of the foot, it makes up the most superficial, medial, delimitating border of the longitudinal arch. It lies over the medial, superficial layer of the flexor digitorum brevis.

Insertion: Medial side of the base of the proximal phalanx of the big toe.

Action

Abducts and supports flexion of the proximal phalanx of the big toe.

Signs of weakness: Hallux valgus and a dropped navicular bone.

Test

Stabilization: On the forefoot.

Test contact: On the medial or tibial portion of the proximal phalanx of the big toe.

Patient: Attempts to abduct the toe in a tibial direction.

Examiner: Carefully, and without too great a pressure, resists the movement by pushing the toe in a fibular direction into adduction.

The ability to perform this movement is difficult for most people.

Myofascial syndrome

Cause for compression: The branches of the medial plantar nerve supplying the intrinsic foot muscles can be compressed by the abductor hallucis when trigger points are present in the muscles.

Frequently found associated disorders

Plantar fasciitis: This painful disorder can be quite debilitating and is most probably due to micro-tears in the plantar fascia. Micro-tearing may be caused by a general hypertonia of the muscles inserting into the fascia; this includes the abductor hallucis.

Compression weakness: Tarsal tunnel syndrome.

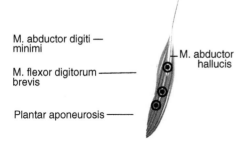

M. abductor digiti — minimi

M. flexor digitorum — brevis

Plantar aponeurosis ——

—M. abductor hallucis

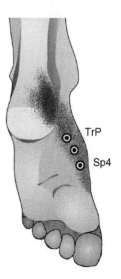

TrP

Sp4

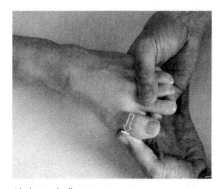

Abductor hallucis test

Motor function innervation: Medial plantar nerve (from the tibial nerve); L5, S1

Anatomy

Origin: The tuberculum of the trapezoid bone, the flexor retinaculum and, in some, the tuberculum of the trapezium bone.

Course: Lying radial to the adductor and the opponens pollicis, the muscle runs lateral and distal.

Insertion: At the radial side of the base of the proximal phalanx of the thumb.

Action

Abduction of the thumb to a point perpendicular to the surface of the palm. From the fully supinated hand, whereby the palm is facing up, the thumb is raised away from the palm.

Signs of weakness: A reduced ability to abduct the thumb noted by difficulty in moving the thumb away from the index finger and in opening the hand fully.

Test

Position: Complete abduction of the thumb by moving it to a point away from and perpendicular to the palm.

Test contact: Must be made very specifically to the anterior or palmar edge of the proximal phalanx of the thumb.

Patient: Attempts to keep the thumb elevated away from the palm by pressing it further into abduction.

Examiner: Carefully resists by pushing the thumb downwards into adduction, towards the index finger.

Test errors, precautions: This test is more difficult to perform than what might be thought at first glance. Asking the patient to raise the thumb from the palm usually results in a combination of extension and abduction. In fact, in cases of weakness, the patient will attempt only to extend the thumb. Even slight errors in examiner contact on the thumb will allow the patient to compensate for weakness. Examiner contact on the thumb from the radial side of the hand is more prone to error as there is a tendency to push on the lateral aspect of the thumb rather than the palmer. Contacting the lateral aspect will place resistance against the extensor muscles. Also, avoid causing pain if the patient has rhizarthrosis (carpometacarpal arthritis of the thumb).

Frequently found associated disorders

The muscle is involved in many thumb related injuries.

Compression weakness: Carpal tunnel and high median nerve entrapment syndromes. The abductor pollicis brevis is better suited for evaluation of carpal tunnel syndrome than the classic opponens pollicis test. Comparing the abductor pollicis longus to the abductor pollicis brevis, a differential diagnosis may be made. The longus, innervated by the radial nerve, is not influenced by entrapment of the median nerve at the carpal tunnel. The abductor pollicis brevis is and, thus, provides the examiner with a simple clinical procedure.

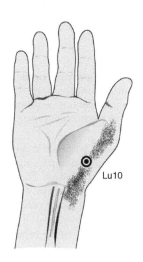

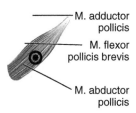

M. adductor pollicis

M. flexor pollicis brevis

M. abductor pollicis

Lu10

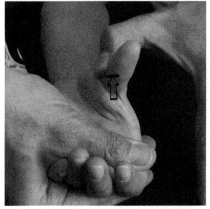

Abductor pollicis brevis test

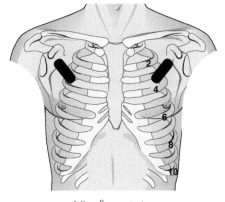

NL reflex anterior

Motor function innervation: Median nerve, C6, C7

Anatomy

Origin: Distal to the origin or the supinator muscle, on the dorsal surface of the ulna, the interosseous membrane and middle third of the dorsal surface of the radius.

Course: Runs in a posterior to anterior direction with the tendon passing over the styloid process of the radius. The tendons of the extensor pollicis longus, extensor pollicis brevis and abductor pollicis longus are visible and palpable.

Insertion: Radial side of the base of the 1st metacarpal bone.

Action

Radial abduction and extension of the 1st metacarpal bone, as if to make a 'karate chop' hand. Radial abduction of the wrist occurs when the thumb is the fixed point. Helps the abductor brevis in palmar abduction of thumb by moving it away from and perpendicular to the palm.

Signs of weakness: Difficulty in radial abduction of the thumb.

Test

Position: The patient flexes the proximal and terminal phalanxes, then extends the thumb by sliding it into extension.

Stabilization: By grasping the hand from the ulnar side, controlling the position of the palm.

Test contact: To the radial surface of the head of the 1st metacarpal.

Patient: Attempts to keep the thumb in abduction by pulling it more radially. The thumb should assume the 'karate chop' position.

Examiner: Pushes the thumb in the direction of palmar adduction.

Test errors, precautions: The contact area is frequently painful due to rhizarthrosis. Pain might falsify the test.

Frequently found associated disorders

Tendovaginitis (tenosynovitis) and trigger point activation, as can develop with excessive poling during skiing.

Compression weakness: Supinator syndrome, narrowing of the upper thoracic outlet.

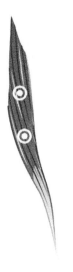

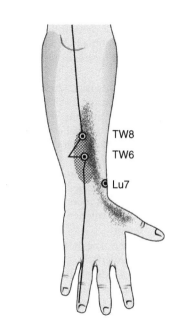

TW8
TW6
Lu7

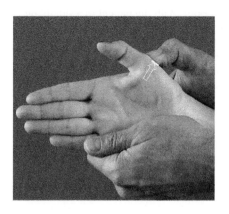

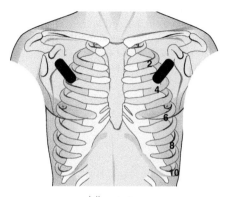

NL anterior

Motor function innervation: Radial nerve, C6, C7, C8

Anatomy

Origin: Pectineus: From the pectineal line of the pubis as far as the pubic tubercle.

Adductor longus: Along the anterior surface of the pubic bone (at the transition of the pubic crest) to the symphysis pubis.

Adductor brevis: Along the lateral surface of the ramus to the inferior aspect of the pubic bone.

Adductor magnus (anterior fibres): From the ramus and inferior parts of the pubic bone and the ramus of the ischium.

Adductor magnus (posterior fibres): The ischial tuberosity.

Course: For the pectineus, adductor brevis and adductor longus as well as the anterior fibres of the adductor magnus: All fibres run from the superior, medial aspect of the femur to the distal, inferior (and somewhat posteriorly) aspect.

Posterior fibres of the adductor magnus: Superiorly from the posterior and medial aspect of the femur to a more distal insertion on both the anterior and medial aspects of the femur.

Insertion: Pectineus: Pectineal line at its most distal point anteriorly.

Adductor longus: Middle third of the linea aspera of the femur more anterior and caudal to the pectineus.

Adductor brevis: From the distal two-thirds of the pectineal line and proximal half of the linea aspera; between the pectineus, adductor longus and adductor magnus.

Adductor magnus: At an area distal to the lesser trochanter along the linea aspera, the adductor tubercle. This insertion is the most posterior of all the divisions.

Action

All muscle divisions: Adduction of the hip joint.

Flexion of the hip joint: Pectineus, adductor brevis, adductor longus and a small part of the anterior fibres of the adductor magnus.

Medial rotation of the hip joint: Pectineus, adductor longus and brevis as well as the anterior fibres of the adductor magnus.

Extension of the hip joint: Posterior fibres of the adductor magnus – the ischiocrural aspect.

During gait: The muscles are active as stabilizers not as prime movers.

The adductor longus is active slightly before the stance phase, during, and for a short time after the toe-off phase (Travell and Simons 1992).

The adductor magnus is active during the entire stance phase, from heel strike until toe off.

The adductor magnus is active when ascending, but not when descending stairs.

Signs of weakness: When standing the pelvis shifts to the opposite side of weakness. Genu varum: A bow-legged deformity is also a possibility.

Test

General adductor muscle test (all divisions) (Kendall and Kendall 1983).

Position: With the patient in a side-lying position, the adductor muscles on the lower leg are tested.

Stabilization: Support the upper leg (the one not being tested) in about 45° abduction.

M. pectineus

M. adductor brevis

M. adductor longus

M. adductor magnus

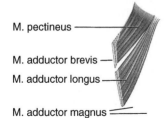

M. adductor magnus, cranial fibres

M. adductor magnus, middle fibres

M. adductor magnus, caudal fibres

M. pectineus, M. adductor longus

M. adductor magnus

M. pectineus and
M. adductor longus
removed

M. adductor magnus
cranial fibres

M. adductor brevis

M. adductor magnus
middle fibres

M. adductor magnus
ischiocrural fibres

M. adductor longus

M. adductor brevis

M. adductor magnus, middle fibres

M. adductor magnus, caudal (ischiocrural) fibres

M. adductor brevis

Adductors viewed from medial

Testing hand position and contact: To the distal, medial thigh, close to the knee of the leg being tested.

Patient: Adducts the lower leg about 20° by lifting it up towards the leg being supported by the examiner.

Examiner: Resists the adduction by attempting to press the lower leg down towards the table, into abduction.

Test in the supine position

Position: The leg not being tested is shifted laterally by abducting it to about 30° while the leg being tested is adducted to about 20° by shifting it medially. No rotation of the legs should be allowed.

Patient: Contracts by approximating the legs in a direction of adduction.

Examiner: Tries to separate the legs by keeping the non-tested leg fixed and pulling the tested leg in a direction of abduction.

Test of the m. adductor longus/m. pectineus (modified Beardall (1981) test)

Position: In the supine position the leg being tested is flexed at the hip to about 30° and the knee is kept in extension. The leg is then internally rotated and adducted so that it moves over the opposite leg and knee to a point of about 30–40° adduction.

Stabilization: Medially on the contralateral lower leg.

Test contact: On the medial, anterior aspect of the distal leg.

Patient: Pulls the legs together into adduction and slight flexion while maintaining medial rotation.

Examiner: Attempts to abduct the legs by pulling them apart.

Test of the m. adductor brevis

Position: Supine.

Stabilization: The non-tested leg is abducted to about 20° and held in place by the examiner. The tested leg is flexed 10–15° at the hip, adducted to about 20° and internally rotated.

Patient: Contracts by pulling the leg into adduction and slight flexion.

Examiner: Pulls in a direction of abduction and slight extension, trying to separate the legs.

Test of the adductor magnus, proximal fibres

Position: Supine.

Stabilization: The non-tested leg is abducted to about 20° and held in place by the examiner. The tested leg is adducted about 20° with no additional flexion, extension or rotation.

Patient: Pulls the legs together into adduction.

Examiner: Pulls in a direction of abduction and slight extension, trying to separate the legs.

Test of the distal, 'ischiocrural' fibres of the adductor magnus

Position: With the patient prone, the non-tested leg is abducted 20° and stabilized by holding firmly in place. The tested leg is extended 15° and adducted 15°.

Test contact: On the medial, dorsal aspect of the lower leg.

Patient: With the knee held in extension, pulls the leg medially into adduction and slight extension.

Examiner: Resists by pulling the leg into abduction and slight flexion.

Testing errors, precautions: Lack of stabilization of the pelvis on the table and imprecise resistance vectors. Should the direction of resistance (vector) by the examiner not be made with exact precision, other fibres and synergistic muscles will be allowed to enter into the test.

Myofascial syndrome

Stretch test: With the patient supine and the leg in extension, it is then abducted and slightly flexed by the examiner to observe the length and tonus of the adductor magnus. The leg is abducted and kept in extension for observing the elongation capacity and tonus of the pectineus, adductor longus and adductor brevis.

PIR: From either of the above stretch positions, the patient holds an inspiration for 10 s and slowly adducts the leg. In the relaxation phase the patient exhales while the examiner abducts the leg by bringing it back to the stretch position and then a bit further, adding a component of extension or flexion for the respective muscles.

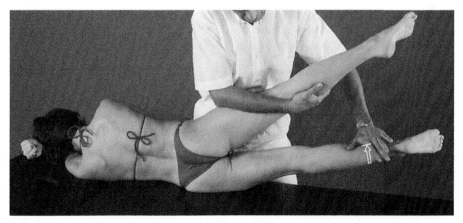

Kendall's general adductor test: the pectineus, adductor longus, adductor brevis and the superior fibres of the adductor magnus are tested by increased flexion and medial rotation of the leg, while the ischiocrural fibres of the adductor magnus are tested by extension of the leg

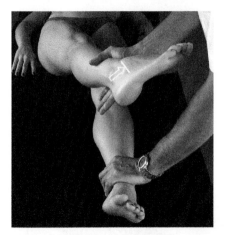

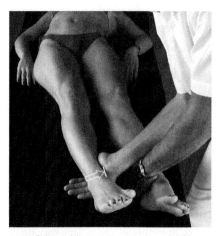

Pectineus and adductor longus test   Test of the adductor magnus, cranial fibres

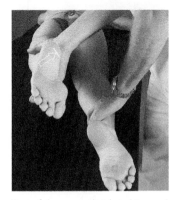

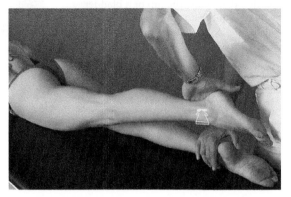

Test of the more distal, ischiocrural fibres of the adductor magnus.

Test of the ischicrural fibres of the adductor magnus, lateral perspective. The hand position shown in the left picture is more ergonomic.

As the adductors are also medial rotators and flexors of the leg, the Patrick (or Faber) position is made on the supine patient by placing the heel on the opposite knee so that the legs make a figure four. This is a good starting position for post-isometric relaxation. During inspiration the patient lifts the knee while the examiner lightly presses the knee down towards the table.

Causes for compression: In certain individuals, a narrowing of the adductor canal by shortening of, and trigger points in, the adductor magnus may compress the femoral artery. The saphenous nerve, providing sensory input to the medial aspect of the lower leg and foot, also runs through the canal. Compression causes dysaesthesia in those areas.

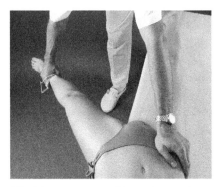

PIR of the pectineus, adductor longus, brevis and magnus, and cranial fibres. Elongation phase

Frequently found associated disorders

Chronic instability of the sacroiliac (SI) joint (Leaf 1996) may cause trigger point development in the adductors with chronic pain in the area of the medial thigh. Athletes may develop forearm problems as a result of reactive patterns between the muscles in the two areas (Goodheart 1976, 1979). Following adductor muscle contraction a prolonged inhibition of the contralateral wrist extensors may be noted (Shafer, verbal information).

Compression weakness: The obturator nerve may be compromised as it passes through the obturator canal. This may be as a result of hypertonicity of the obturator muscles, damage to the hip or a bladder fixation as understood in visceral osteopathy.

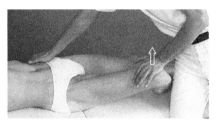

PIR of a very shortened pectineus, and superior fibres of the adductor longus, brevis and magnus. Contraction phase

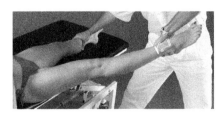

PIR of the adductor magnus and ischiocrural fibres. Contraction phase

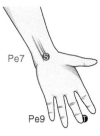

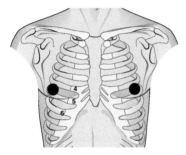

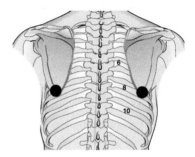

NL anterior   NL posterior

Motor function innervation:
Pectineus: Femoral nerve, obturator nerve, L2, L3, L4
Adductor brevis, adductor longus: Obturator nerve, L2, L3, L4
Adductor magnus: Obturator nerve, L2, L3, L4 and sciatic nerve, L4, L5
Visceroparietal segment (TS line): L5
Rib pump: Intercostal space, costotransverse joint 1, 2, 4, 5, 7
Meridian: Pericardium
Organ: Gonads
Nutrients: Vitamins A, B3, C, E, PUFA, Mg, Se Zn

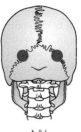

NV

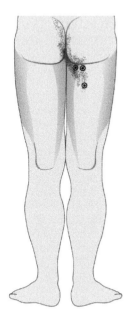

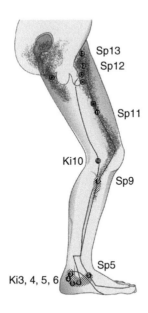

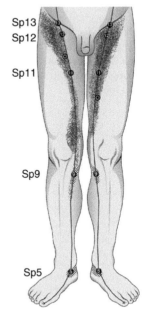

Trigger points in the ischiocrural part of the adductor magnus and pain radiation pattern into the perineum, rectum and prostate (also see next figure)

Trigger points near the kidney and spleen meridians. Effective distal points lie in an area around the medial ankle

Trigger points of the pectineus, adductor longus and brevis on the right leg. Trigger points of the cranial part of the adductor magnus on the left leg

M. adductor hallucis

Anatomy

Origin: Oblique head: Cuboid bone, lateral cuneiform bone, base of the 2nd to 4th metatarsals and tendonal sheath of the peroneus longus.

Transverse head: Capsular ligaments of the metatarsophalangeal joint of the 3rd to 5th toes and deep transverse metatarsal ligament.

Course: The oblique head runs obliquely from posterior to the common insertion. The transverse head traverses from lateral to medial to the common insertion. Both heads lie in the middle layer of the plantar muscles. The deep layer is formed by the plantar interossei and the most superficial layer by the abductor hallucis, abductor digiti minimi and flexor hallucis brevis.

Insertion: On the lateral side of the base of the proximal phalanx of the big toe together with the medial tendon of the flexor hallucis brevis.

Action

Abducts and supports flexion of the proximal phalanx of the big toe.

Signs of weakness: A drooping of the longitudinal and transverse arch of the foot.

Test

Test contact: On the fibular aspect at the base of the proximal phalanx of the big toe.

Patient: Attempts to keep the toe in adduction by pressing it in a fibular direction.

Examiner: Resists into abduction by carefully pulling or pushing the big toe in a tibial (medial) direction.

It is very difficult for the patient to coordinate the contraction of the great toe during this test.

Frequently found associated disorders

Splayfoot, characterized by a dropped arch, flattening and spreading out of the foot.

Compression weakness: Tarsal tunnel syndrome.

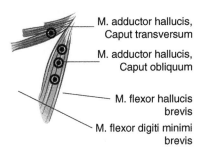

M. adductor hallucis,
Caput transversum

M. adductor hallucis,
Caput obliquum

M. flexor hallucis
brevis

M. flexor digiti minimi
brevis

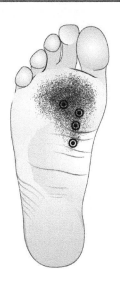

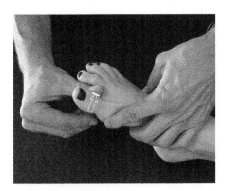

Adductor hallucis test

Motor function innervation: Medial plantar nerve (from the tibial nerve): S1, S2

Anatomy

Origin: Oblique head: Base of the 2nd and 3rd metacarpals and the capitate bone.

Transverse head: Palmar surface of the 3rd metacarpal bone.

Course: The fibres converge to end on the proximal phalanx of the thumb, running more medial and distal to the opponens pollicis.

Insertion: Oblique head: dorsal aponeurosis of the thumb.

Transverse head: Ulnar side of the base of the proximal phalanx of the thumb.

Action

It primarily adducts the proximal phalanx of the thumb by approximating it to the palm of the hand. Understanding the action of the intrinsic muscles of the thumb is not always a clear, straightforward task. Movement of the thumb is linked to the plane of the hand, not the body. Therefore, abduction and adduction must be related to the palm. Abduction will bring the thumb up and away from the hand so that it is perpendicular to the palm. Adduction will bring it down from the perpendicular position so that it touches the palm. Therefore, if the wrist and hand are put into supination so that the palm is pointing upwards, the thumb will be brought down towards the index finger. The muscle also aids in opposition of the thumb with the little finger and in bringing the thumb to the side of the index finger.

Signs of weakness: Gripping small objects like pencils or pens and using chopsticks. The thumb cannot be pressed firmly on the index finger with the fist closed.

Test

Position: The thumb is kept in extension and placed on the palmar aspect of the 2nd metacarpal (index finger). Arriving at this point is not easy as most patients will flex the thumb, bringing the flexor pollicis brevis into the test. More often than not, the examiner must place the thumb in the correct start position for the patient.

Stabilization: Approaching from the ulnar side, the hand is grasped, keeping the palm in supination. The testing hand must hold the thumb so that the two more distal joints are held in extension.

Test contact: Approaching from the ulnar side of the hand, the fingers slide between the thumb and the index finger to contact the dorsal ulnar side of the thumb. The thumb of the examiner may be used to keep the proximal joints of the patients thumb in extension.

Patient: Keeping the thumb extended, draws it towards the index finger.

Examiner: Resists by pulling the thumb away from the palm and index finger.

A simple, but less specific test may also be made. A piece of paper is placed between the extended thumb and the palmer surface of the index finger. The patient is instructed to hold the paper in place and resist its extraction by the examiner.

Test errors, precautions: Thumb flexion is the most common compensatory movement during testing. The adductor pollicis has a synergistic effect on thumb flexion. This is easily observed during the test by the patient continually flexing the thumb while attempting to adduct, if there is weakness. Therefore the test vector must be accurately observed as described. No cupping of the hand is allowed during the test otherwise the muscle cannot be differentiated from the opponens pollicis. Keeping the palm flat is clinically important as the muscles have different innervations. The ulnar nerve innervates the adductor brevis and the median the opponens pollicis.

Myofascial syndrome

Stretch test: The thumb is extended in dorsal direction to the point of elastic restriction. No differentiation from hypertonic abductor pollicis brevis, opponens and flexor pollicis muscles is possible.

PIR: From the stretch position and against gentle resistance by the examiner, the patient slowly contracts the muscle to bring the thumb into adduction towards the index finger. In the relaxation phase, the examiner gradually abducts the thumb, returning it to the starting position;

applying a further, slight stretch at the endpoint of elastic restriction.

Frequently found associated disorders

Weakness of the muscle occurs with entrapments of the ulnar nerve as found in pisiform hamate syndrome. In more severe cases, a functional weakness may be apparent and, in the thenar area, a loss of mass will signal muscle atrophy. Individual testing of the opponens and adductor pollicis will allow for differentiation between carpal tunnel and pisiform hamate syndromes.

Clinically, the adductor pollicis may have even greater importance as a specific indicator muscle for C8 and T1 nerve lesions.

Compression weakness: Ulnar tunnel and pisiform hamate syndromes.

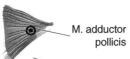

M. adductor pollicis

M. opponens pollicis

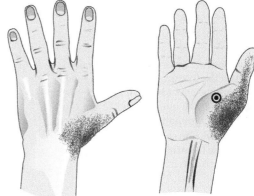

Motor function innervation:
Ulnar nerve, C8, T1

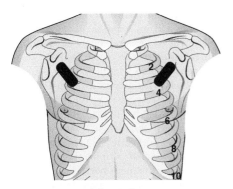

NL anterior

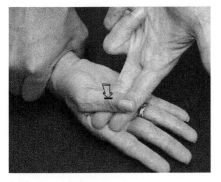

Adductor pollicis test

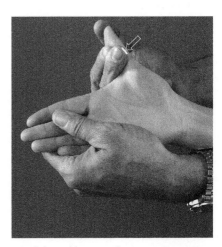

PIR of the adductor pollicis – contraction phase

M. biceps brachii

Anatomy

Origin: Long head: On the glenoid tubercle of the scapula.
Short head: On the coracoid process together with the coracobrachialis muscle.
Course: The tendon of the long head runs through the intertubercular sulcus and over the head of the humerus, remaining extra-capsular along its route.
Insertion: With the common tendon at the radial tuberosity.

Action

Both divisions flex the elbow joint and supinate the forearm. The long head aids in flexing the shoulder joint and helps with abduction of the humerus, while the short head helps with adduction of the humerus.
Signs of weakness: The patient tends to pronate the forearm when flexing the elbow.

Test

Position: The elbow is flexed 80° and supinated.
Stabilization: At the base of the elbow.
Test contact: To the distal forearm.
Patient: Attempts to bend the elbow using maximum strength.
Examiner: Resists trying to extend the elbow joint.

Testing the long head of the biceps (proximal fibres)

Position: With the patient supine, the humerus is flexed 45° and abducted about 20°. Thereafter, the forearm is supinated and flexed about 45° to 60° at the elbow. The forearm will be almost vertical to the floor. The patient makes a fist keeping the wrist in a straight line with the forearm.
Stabilization: On the anterior aspect of the shoulder, should this be necessary. In the seated position, stabilization might be more important than in the supine.
Test contact: On the top of the patient's fist with one hand if the other is stabilizing the shoulder and two hands if not.
Patient: Without flexing the elbow any further, pushes the fist upward.
Examiner: Resists by pushing the fist down towards the table, in a vector that passes through the elbow following the arc of movement of the arm about the shoulder.
Test errors, precautions: Allowing the elbow to change flexion angle and too little supination of the forearm.

Myofascial syndrome

Stretch test: The elbow is extended and the forearm pronated. The muscle is passively stretched through shoulder extension by bringing the arm behind the body.
PIR: The examiner keeps the muscle in the extreme stretch position by holding the shoulder and the arm in extension. The patient makes a very slight contraction of the biceps by attempting to flex the shoulder and elbow while the examiner keeps the extremity in extension. This is followed by the relaxation phase where the examiner, predominantly at the shoulder, gently increases the limb extension.

Frequently found associated disorders

Tendinitis of the tendon of the long head is often seen and, on occasion, luxation of the tendon will occur. A relatively common pain, noted only in the right shoulder and not associated with the biceps, is caused by an open ileocecal valve. The neurolymphatic reflex zone for the valve lies along the tendon of the long head.
Compression weakness: Root lesions of C5 and C6 at intervertebral foramen levels C4/5 and C5/6 and peripheral entrapment of the musculocutaneus nerve may ensue as it passes through the coracobrachialis muscle.

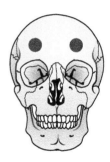

NV

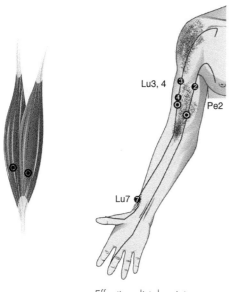

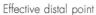

Lu3, 4

Pe2

Lu7

Effective distal point

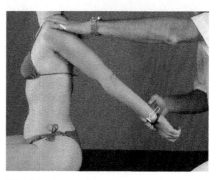

PIR of the biceps brachii

Motor function innervation:
Musculocutaneous nerve, C5, C6
Rib pump: Intercostal space,
costotransverse joint 7, 9
Meridian: Stomach
Organ: Stomach
Nutrients: Ca, Mg, Fe, vit. B5, PUFA,
phosphatase

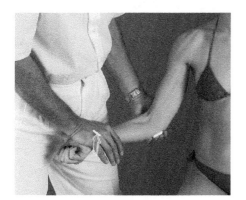

Testing the function of the elbow flexion

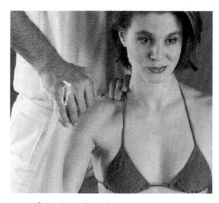

Test of the long head

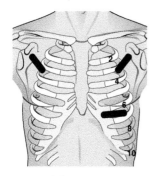

NL posterior

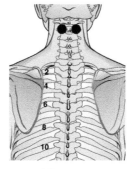

NL anterior

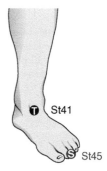

St41

St45

M. brachialis

Anatomy

Origin: At a point below the deltoid tuberosity, on the distal two-thirds of the anterior shaft of the humerus, and the medial and lateral intermuscular septum.

Course: From superior to inferior, lying below the biceps brachii; it can be felt medially and laterally at the distal half between the biceps muscle and the humerus bone.

Insertion: At the ulnar tuberosity.

Action

Pure flexion of the elbow joint.

Test

Position: The elbow is flexed to 80° and the forearm held half way between pronation and supination so that the thumb of the hand is up. This differentiates the test from that of the biceps brachii where the test is made in full supination. The brachialis, though, cannot be easily separated from the brachioradialis during testing. The brachioradialis is tested as above according to Kendall and Kendall (1983) and Walther (2000). But according to Beardall (1983), the brachioradialis test made with full pronation of the forearm distinguishes it from the brachialis.

Stabilization: At the elbow.

Test contact: To the distal forearm at a point roughly corresponding to the strength of the patient.

Patient: Bends the elbow with maximum strength.

Examiner: Resists pushing the elbow into extension and following the normal arc of motion as the forearm moves about the elbow.

Test errors, precautions: Permitting supination of the forearm and poor elbow stabilization that allows changes of the angle of the humerus at the shoulder.

Myofascial syndrome

Stretch test: The shoulder is flexed to relax the long head of the biceps, the forearm is supinated and the elbow put into maximum extension.

PIR: Is only effective when there is severe shortening of the muscle such that elbow extension is limited. From the stretch position, the patient is instructed to inspire and slowly flex the elbow against resistance for 10 s. In the relaxation phase, the patient breathes out while the examiner gently returns the limb to the stretch position.

Cause for compression: The superficial cutaneous branch of the radial nerve as it courses down the humerus can become irritated, usually following traumatic insult, and will lead to numbness or pain on the back of the thumb.

Frequently found associated disorders

The muscle should be evaluated for compensatory reactions, trigger points and reactive patterns following any injury involving the elbow or the wrist.

Compression weakness: Entrapment of the musculocutaneus nerve as it passes through the coracobrachialis muscle and restrictions involving the C6 root at the C5/C6 intervertebral foramen (Patten 1998).

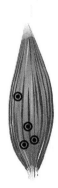

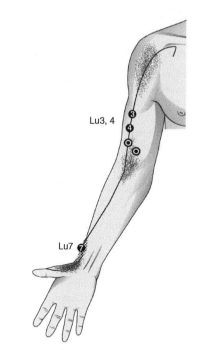

Effective distal point Lu7

Lu3, 4

Lu7

Motor function innervation: Musculocutaneous nerve, C5, C6
Meridian: Stomach
Organ: Stomach
Nutrients: Ca, Mg, Fe, vit. B5, PUFA, phosphatase

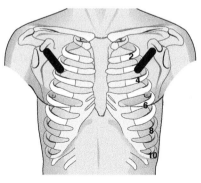

NL anterior

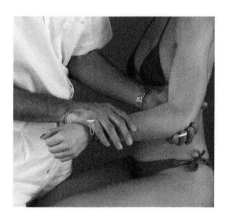

Brachialis test

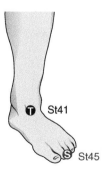

St41

St45

M. brachioradialis

Anatomy

Origin: On the lateral margin of the humerus, as far as the insertion of the deltoid, and on the lateral intermuscular septum.

Course: From superior to inferior, it is the most radial (lateral) of the elbow flexors.

Insertion: On the radius, proximal to the styloid process.

Action

Powerful elbow flexion with forearm pronation and aids in returning the forearm from either pronation or supination to the mid-position.

Signs of weakness: The arm hangs extended at the elbow like a limp rope.

Test

Position: The elbow is flexed 75° and the forearm held in the mid-position between pronation and supination so that the thumb points up (Walther 1981, Kendall and Kendall 1983). According to Beardall (1983) the brachioradialis will be the prime mover with the forearm in full pronation, while the brachialis muscle is best tested in neutral position as described above.

Stabilization: At the elbow.

Test contact: To the distal forearm.

Patient: Flexes the forearm against resistance by the examiner.

Examiner: Resists by pushing the forearm into extension following the natural arc of motion about the elbow.

Test errors, precautions: Inadequate stabilization of the elbow.

Myofascial syndrome

Stretch test: The elbow is extended and supported in that position, followed by forearm pronation and the hand put in full ulnar adduction. This position should be able to evoke pain due to trigger points.

PIR: Not very effective for this muscle as elbow extension is normally restricted. Trigger points and increased tension will almost always occur in conjunction with dysfunction of the extensors of the hand and fingers and they should be treated at the same time.

Frequently found associated disorders

Symptoms mimicking 'epicondylitis' can arise from trigger points in the muscle with referred pain radiating out laterally.

Compression weakness: The brachioradialis is the indicator muscle for lesions of the C6 root emanating from the C5/C6 intervertebral foramen (Patten 1998).

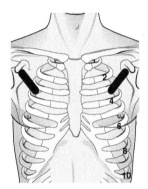

NL anterior

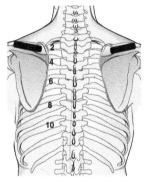

NL posterior

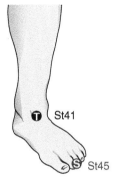

St41

St45

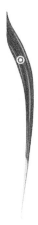

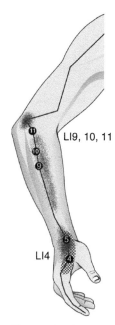

LI9, 10, 11

LI4

Effective distal points

Motor function innervation: Radial nerve, C5, C6
Rib pump: Intercostal space, costotransverse joint 4, 5
Meridian: Stomach
Organ: Stomach
Nutrients: Ca, Mg, Fe, vit. B5, PUFA, phosphatase

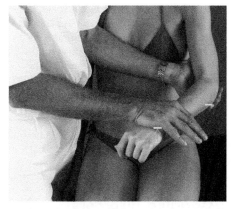

Brachioradialis test

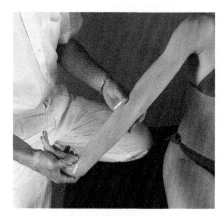

PIR of the brachioradialis

Anatomy

Origin: Together with the short head of the biceps at the coracoid process.

Course: Runs from superior to inferior, inserting below the tendon of the short head of the biceps.

Insertion: In the middle of the humerus at the crest of the lesser tubercle.

Action

Flexion and adduction of the humerus.

Signs of weakness: Difficulty in touching the back of the head and neck as when combing the hair.

Test

Position: Flexion of the shoulder to 45° and abduction to about 45°. An incremental lateral rotation of 10° is added with forearm supination and full flexion of the elbow in order to maximize shortening of the synergistic biceps brachii.

Stabilization: At the shoulder.

Test contact: From the medial side, on the patient's upper arm, just above the bent elbow. Alternatively, when the patient is strong and the thumb of the examiner weak, contact may be made externally, on the forearm. This last contact may even further take the biceps out of the test.

Patient: Flexes the upper arm against resistance by pushing the elbow up and towards the head, adding a slight adduction component.

Examiner: Resists by pushing the elbow down to extend the shoulder and slightly outward, away from the body to bring the arm into abduction. Due to extremely powerful biceps and deltoid synergism, it is very important to precisely follow the arc of motion of the arm produced by coracobrachialis contraction alone. Too great an abduction resistance will introduce the pectoralis muscles into the test and too little external rotation will introduce the biceps and anterior deltoid into the test.

With strong patients, especially athletes, it is better to make contact from above, over the forearm, as described above.

Test errors, precautions: Insufficient or too great an abduction component. Too little external rotation and shoulder flexion greater than 45°. With the elbow too elevated, the origin and insertion are brought into alignment that effectively eliminates any capacity to further flexion.

Alternative testing: In situations where there are no clear test responses, the starting position may be elevated to a point of about 70°. Certainly this position will take the biceps out of the test, but care must be taken so that the elevation does not pass the level of the coracoid process, otherwise the anterior deltoid will be the prime mover.

Compression weakness

Lesions of the C6 root from the C5/6 intervertebral foramen leads to weakness of the coracobrachialis muscle (Patten 1998). Entrapments at the thoracic inlet (scalenus and costoclavicular syndromes) may also weaken the muscle.

Myofascial syndrome

Stretch test: The humerus is extended, maximally abducted and laterally rotated. Isolation of the coracobrachialis from the biceps or even the pectoralis, pars clavicularis is not possible.

PIR: The patient is supine with the arm in the above stretch position and instructed to contract the muscle against only the weight of the arm. In the relaxation phase, the arm is allowed, again using only it's own weight, to slowly return to the stretch position.

Cause for compression: Leaf (1996) has described a situation whereby hypertonus of the muscle can lead to entrapment of the musculocutaneus nerve. This will be especially noted when working with the hands above the level of the head for long periods of time. Travell and Simons (1983) controversially write that this rarely seems to occur clinically. Symptoms would include weakness of the biceps brachii, brachialis and paraesthesia of the radial side of the forearm.

Frequently found associated disorders

Functional inhibition is frequently linked to hypertonus of the synergistic deltoid and vice versa.

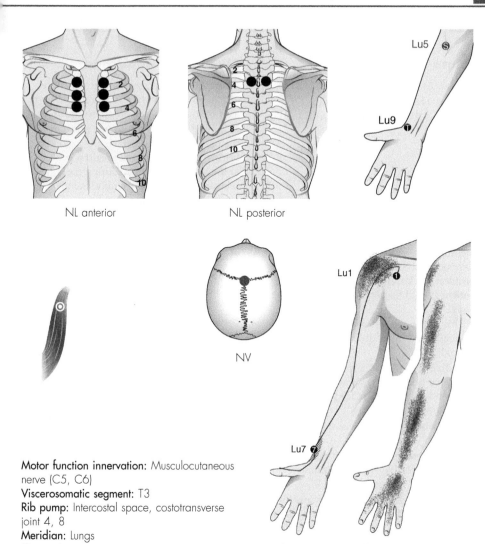

NL anterior

NL posterior

NV

Referred pain and effective distal point

Motor function innervation: Musculocutaneous nerve (C5, C6)
Viscerosomatic segment: T3
Rib pump: Intercostal space, costotransverse joint 4, 8
Meridian: Lungs
Organ: Lungs
Nutrients: Vitamins C and E, beta-carotene, selenium, N-acetylcysteine (NAC)

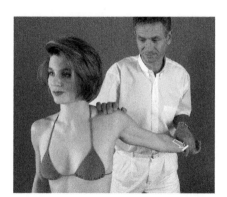

PIR of the coracobrachialis

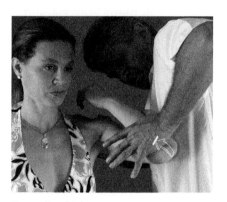

Coracobrachialis test

Anatomy

Origin: At the acromion process.
Course: The fibres run vertically.
Insertion: At the deltoid tuberosity of the humerus.

Action

Together with the other two divisions, abduction of the humerus.

Test

Position: The elbow is flexed to 90° and the humerus, without any imparted rotation, is abducted to 90°. In the test position, the hand and forearm of the patient should be perpendicular to the body.

This is also the test position for the combined test of all divisions of the deltoid.

Stabilization: With the patient seated and the upper body in a neutral position, the free hand is normally placed on the opposite shoulder.

Test contact: Avoiding painful points, at the elbow.

Patient: Attempts to elevate the elbow as hard as possible against examiner resistance.

Examiner: Resists abduction by pushing down on the elbow. It is important that the resistance vector run straight down. No shoulder flexion or extension component must be allowed.

In exceptional cases, the test can be performed with the elbow extended if the power ratio of the patient to the examiner requires the use of a longer lever.

Test errors, precautions: The humerus must be fully abducted to 90° before the test and the test vector must be precisely downward into adduction. No rotation of the humerus should be allowed. An effort should be made not to use the 'long lever' deltoid test unless there is a significant power difference between the examiner and patient. In these cases, greater care must be made to stabilize the patient from body inclination during the test.

Myofascial syndrome

Stretch test: With the patient seated, the arm is brought down and behind the body as if trying to grasp the opposite scapula.

PIR: Starting from the stretch position, the patient slowly contracts the muscle to bring the arm back to the neutral position at the side of the trunk. During the relaxation phase, the examiner gently elongates the muscle by returning it to the position of stretch.

Frequently found associated disorders (all divisions)

If functional weakness is noted bilaterally, it is an indication of micro-fixations at the cervicodorsal junction.

Injury to the deltoid can lead to instability of the acromioclavicular joint. Likewise, injuries to the joint and its ligaments will tend to inhibit the deltoid. Weakness of the deltoid can lead to hypertonus of the upper trapezius and concomitant development of trigger points.

Compression weakness: Lesion of the C5 root leads to weakness of the deltoid together with all the other shoulder abductors (Patten 1998). As well, scalenus, costoclavicular and pectoralis minor syndromes can all lead to weakness. The three brachial plexus compression sites can adversely affect the axillary nerve as it exits the armpit from the posterior fasciculus. Nerve entrapment may also occur distal to the brachial plexus as found in the lateral axillary hiatus syndrome.

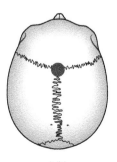

NV

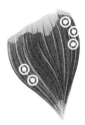

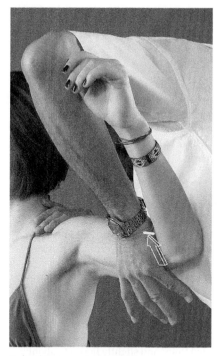

Deltoid test – anterior division

Motor function innervation: Axillary nerve, C4, C5, C6
Viscerosomatic segment (TS line): T3
Rib pump: Intercostal space, costotransverse joint 2, 3, 4, 7, 10
Organ: Lungs, thymus
Nutrients: Vitamins C and E, beta-carotene, selenium, N-acetylcysteine
SRS: Thoracic segments and first two lumbar segments

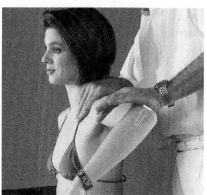

Deltoid test – posterior division

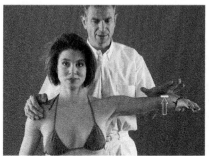

Deltoid test – middle division

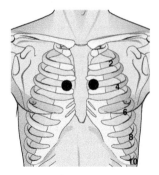

NV anterior

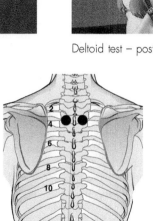

NV posterior

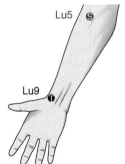

Lu5

Lu9

Anterior division (clavicular part)

Anatomy

Origin: On the acromial third of the clavicle.

Course: Converging from an anterior, superior origin to a posterior, lateral and inferior insertion.

Insertion: At the deltoid tuberosity of the humerus.

Action

Abduction, flexion and medial rotation of the upper arm.

Signs of weakness: A slight lateral rotation in the hanging arm and difficulty in obtaining and maintaining the test position so that other muscles are recruited.

Test

Position: The elbow is flexed to 90°. Then the upper arm is abducted to 90°, laterally rotated to 45° and slightly flexed to about 10°.

Stabilization: On top of and slightly to the back of the patient's shoulder.

Test contact: On the distal upper arm just above the crease of the flexed elbow.

Patient: Presses upward, elevating the arm into abduction and into slight flexion in the direction that is in line with the forearm.

Examiner: Resists the motion by pushing downward and into slight extension in a direction that follows that of the forearm.

Test errors, precautions: As with the middle division, the humerus must be fully abducted and the resistance vector must follow a direction of adduction and extension. Allowing the arm to internally rotate to bring the other divisions into the test.

Myofascial syndrome

Stretch test: Even though this stretch test is not very specific, the seated patient is asked to laterally rotate the arm and extend the shoulder.

PIR: Starting from the above stretch position, the patient slowly contracts the muscle bringing the shoulder and arm to the neutral position. In the relaxation phase, the examiner gently stretches the muscle by bringing the arm and shoulder back to the start position.

Posterior division (spinal part)

Anatomy

Origin: Lateral two-thirds of the spine of the scapula.

Course: Converges laterally from a posterior, superior origin to an anterior, inferior insertion.

Insertion: In a common insertion on the deltoid tuberosity of the humerus.

Action

Extension, lateral rotation and abduction of the humerus.

Signs of weakness: Slight medial rotation of the hanging arm.

Test

Position: Similar to the above, the patient starts by bending the elbow to 90°, followed by placing the humerus into 90° of abduction. The difference is made by medially rotating the humerus to 45° and slightly extending the shoulder to about 10°.

Stabilization: To the superior and anterior shoulder.

Test contact: On the elbow, from behind and above, slightly lateral to and over the olecranon fossa of the humerus.

Patient: Attempting to follow the angle of the internally rotated forearm, presses the elbow back and up so as to extend the arm.

If a longer lever is required, greater care must be taken with the posterior than with the anterior and middle divisions. The posterior division, in most individuals, is not very strong and internal rotation of the humerus puts the elbow in a weaker position to resist unwanted flexion. In cases where there is a weak triceps, the long lever test might not be possible.

Test errors, precautions: The humerus must be fully abducted before the test and the testing vector must be accurately followed. The patient must be prevented from laterally rotating the arm and tilting the body to the opposite side in order to recruit the m. supraspinatus.

Myofascial syndrome

Stretch test: The arm of the seated patient is adducted fully by drawing the arm slightly downward and as far as it will go across the chest.

PIR: Starting from the stretch position, the patient slowly contracts the muscle to return the arm to the neutral position. This is followed by the relaxation phase where the examiner gently elongates the muscle by bringing the arm back to the starting point.

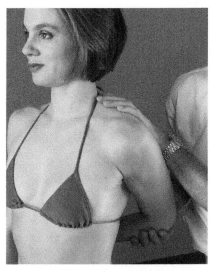

PIR deltoid, middle and anterior divisions

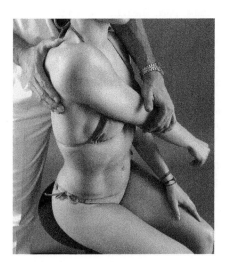

PIR deltoid posterior division

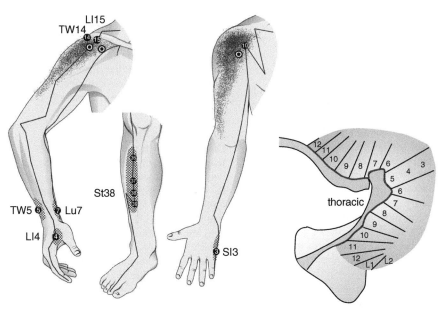

Effective distal points

SR zones for all divisions of the deltoid

Anatomy

Origin: Sternal part: On the medial surface of the xiphoid process.

Costal part: On the medial surface of the six bottom ribs.

Lumbar part: The right crus (right side of the diaphragm) arises from the 1st to 4th lumbar vertebrae. The left crus has its origin from the 1st to 3rd lumbar verte-brae. The medial arcuate ligament of the diaphragm courses from the 1st lumbar vertebra, over the ilio-psoas muscle, to the costal process of L1. The lateral arcuate ligament passes anterior to the quadratus lumborum muscle and runs from the costal process of L1 to the apex of the 12th rib.

Diaphramatic outlets from the thorax to the abdomen: The hiatus venae cavae is the most anterior of the three and somewhat to the right of the midline.

The oesophageal hiatus is slightly left of the midline and is bordered by the cross-ing fibres of the right and left crus and anterior bodies of the lumbar vertebrae.

Between the right and left crus: Hiatus aorticus.

Insertion: In the central tendon. This is a flat aponeurosis in the middle of the diaphragmatic vault to which run all the muscle fibres.

Action

The diaphragm is the primary muscle of respiration. Contraction of the muscle leads to a lowering of the vault of the diaphragm. The diaphragm strongly influences the pressure differential in the thoracic and abdominal cavities. Because of this it is also important in blood and lymph transport. Together, the right and left crura help to close the cardiac sphincter.

Primarily described in osteopathy, but gaining evermore support from other disciplines, the diaphragm is thought to be one of the main mechanisms for the maintenance of visceral motility as well as the lymphatic flow.

Signs of weakness: Excursion of the thorax on the weak side, abdominal expansion, vital capacity and forced expiratory volume are all reduced.

Diaphragmatic testing and examination procedures

The diaphragm cannot be directly tested with manual muscle testing. The following checks on function can be used.

Snider's test (Walther 2000)

This is a simple screening test. A burning match is held 15 cm in front of the patient's wide open mouth. The flame is held about 10 cm lower than the mouth, as the air flow when exhaling is angled downwards through the upper incisors. The patient is asked to try to blow out the flame with one breath while keeping the mouth wide open. The test can vary according to the exact distance and angle from the mouth as well as the type of match used. Forced expiratory volume measurements are more precise and the instruments, these days, are very economical.

Palpation

The examiner places both hands lightly on the sides of the lower thorax and compares their excursion while the patient breathes in. Diaphragm muscle weakness is indicated by the side with reduced excursion. An increased lateral rotation of the leg on the same side of diaphragmatic weakness is frequently noted. It is believed that this may be caused by a reactive hypertonicity of the psoas related to the weakness of the diaphragm.

TL and challenge

Diaphragm dysfunction is diagnosed using applied kinesiology by TL just below the xyphoid of the sternum. A NIM becomes weak (dysreactive) as a result if there is dysfunction of the diaphragm.

If, after the above challenge, no indicator muscle weakness is evident, the patient is then asked to breathe in and out three or four times while maintaining the TL contact. After this combined challenge, a corresponding weakening of the indicator muscle often occurs when the diaphragm is malfunctioning.

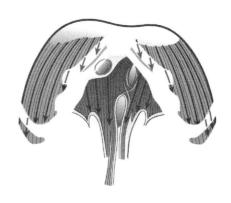

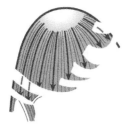

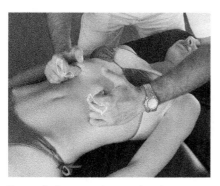

Direct challenge at the costal arch

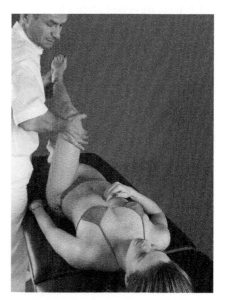

The diaphragm is evaluated with a combination of therapy localization below the xyphoid and respiratory challenge. A weakening (dysreaction) of a NIM will indicate a positive test

Direct challenge

The diaphragm can be directly challenged by contacting underneath the right and left costal arches, simultaneously. The examiner places the ulnar margins of the flat hands deep below the costal arch and applies a traction challenge on the diaphragm. This is done by pushing the hands in a diagonal fashion posteriorly towards the spine and superiorly towards the skull. Again, if there is dysfunction of the diaphragm, as a result of this challenge (provocation), a NIM weakens (becomes dysreactive).

Frequently found associated disorders

Diaphragm dysfunction often occurs when there are mechanical problems within the middle cervicals (C3 to C5) and with micro fixations of the thoracolumbar junction area.

An abnormal diaphragm and disorders of the visceral are almost always linked.

For example, if the liver becomes fixated to the surrounding fascia it will, without a doubt, cause disruption of normal diaphragm movement patterns. In reflux oesophagitis, invariably, the first step must be to normalize diaphragm function. The diaphragmatic crura surround and support the cardiac sphincter and asymmetry within the muscle may easily lead to irritation of the area.

Any disorder involving oxygenation, with an O_2 saturation of less than 98%, must be treated first by normalizing rib and diaphragm function. When the most sensitive structures of the central nervous system (CNS) are functionally disturbed, the quality and quantity of oxygen reaching the brain must be normalized and the diaphragm is crucial to recovery. The importance in maintaining optimum oxygenation of the brain cannot be underestimated.

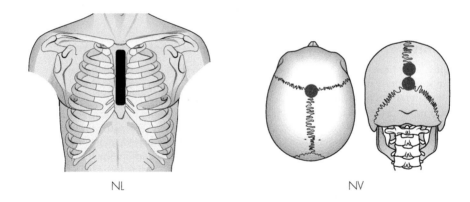

NL   NV

Motor function innervation: Phrenic nerve, C3, C4, C5
Visceroparietal segment (TS line): Between T5 and T6
Meridian: Conception vessel (CV, Ren Mai)

Anatomy

Origin: Long head: Distal third of the lateral supracondylar ridge of the humerus and the lateral intermuscular septum.

Short head: On the lateral epicondyle of the humerus, lateral collateral ligament of the elbow joint and the antebrachial fascia.

Course: Runs superficially between the m. brachioradialis, m. extensor digitorum and the extensor carpi radialis brevis, distally.

Insertion: Long head: Posterior radial aspect of the base of the 2nd metacarpal bone.

Short head: Posterior aspect of the base of the third metacarpal bone.

Action

Extension and radial abduction of the wrist. The longus is also a synergist in elbow flexion.

Signs of weakness: Ulnar adduction of the hand.

Test

Position: The forearm is pronated in the range of 45–80°, followed by extension and radial abduction of the wrist.

Stabilization: On the distal third of the forearm.

Test contact: On the dorsum of the hand, covering its radial aspect, in the area of the 1st and 2nd metacarpals.

Patient: Extends the hand on the wrist by pulling the 1st and 2nd metacarpals upwards and radially.

Examiner: Resists over the radial aspect of the dorsum of the hand, pushing it into flexion and ulnar adduction.

Test errors, precautions: Pain on contact, lack of stabilization of the wrist and forearm, and allowing the extensor carpi ulnaris to enter into the test.

Myofascial syndrome

Stretch test: With the elbow fully extended, the wrist is flexed and adducted to the ulnar side.

PIR: The wrist and arm are held in the stretch position. The patient minimally contracts the muscle against resistance by moving the hand in the direction of extension and radial abduction. For the relaxation phase the examiner returns the hand to the starting point by ulnar adduction and flexion of the wrist. At the end a slight exaggeration of the stretch is made.

Cause for compression: Adverse tension in the brevis portion can lead to irritation of the sensory branch of the radial nerve as it passes through the body of the muscle and lead to dysaesthesia of the back of the hand.

Frequently found associated disorders

Pain that mimics a 'tennis elbow'.

Compression weakness: From the thoracic inlet, radial sulcus, and radial nerve syndrome. Lesions of the C7 root from the C6/7 disc can lead to weakness of the muscle (Patten 1998). Thoracic inlet entrapments stemming from scalene, costoclavicular and coracopectoral syndromes.

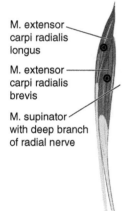

M. extensor carpi radialis longus

M. extensor carpi radialis brevis

M. supinator with deep branch of radial nerve

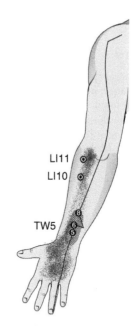

LI11
LI10
TW5

Effective distal point

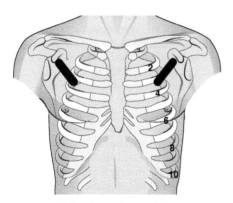

NL anterior

Motor function innervation: Radial nerve, C5, C6, C7
Nutrients: Ca, Mg, Fe, vit. B5, PUFA, phosphatase

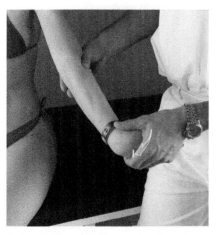

Post isometric relaxation: contraction phase

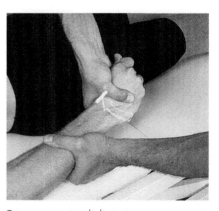

Extensor carpi radialis test

M. extensor carpi ulnaris

Anatomy

Origin: Lateral epicondyle of the humerus, posterior margin of the ulna and antebrachial fascia.

Course: Over the ulnar surface of the forearm, between the extensor digitorum and anconeus (if present) muscles.

Insertion: Ulnar side of the base of the 5th metacarpal bone.

Action

Extension and ulnar adduction hand on the wrist.

Signs of weakness: Radial abduction and flexion of the hand.

Test

Position: The hand is placed into ulnar adduction and extension.

Stabilization: Under the patient's distal forearm in a general, non-specific area.

Test contact: To the dorsum of the hand close to its ulnar aspect, covering the 5th metacarpal bone.

Patient: Presses the hand back and up into ulnar adduction and extension.

Examiner: Resists by pressing the hand into flexion and ulnar abduction.

Test errors, precautions: Pain during the test, inadequate stabilization, a contact placed too far to the radial side and permitting any radial deviation of the hand during testing.

Myofascial syndrome

Stretch test: The elbow is placed in full extension and supported. Then the wrist is flexed and radially abducted.

PIR: From the stretch position, the patient slowly contracts in the direction of extension and ulnar adduction of the hand. In the relaxation phase a gentle stretch is made in the direction of flexion and radial abduction. As radial abduction is not pronounced it is only possible to a minimal extent, during wrist flexion, to stretch the muscle. Other myofascial therapies for treatment of the muscle are more suitable.

Frequently found associated disorders

Pain that mimics a 'tennis elbow'.

Note: For evaluating radial nerve involvement, a group test of the extensor carpi radialis and ulnaris together, may be made. Stabilization at the distal forearm remains the same. The patient extends the wrist straight back, without any radial or ulnar deviation, and presses in the direction of extension. The examiner resists the movement, following the arc of motion of the hand as moves into flexion.

Compression weakness: Lesions of the C7 root from the C6/7 disc can lead to weakness of the muscle (Patten 1998). As with the radialis, thoracic inlet, radial sulcus entrapment, radial nerve and supinator syndromes, will all cause some degree of muscle weakness.

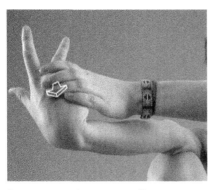

Postisometric relaxation as self treatment

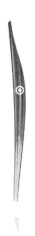

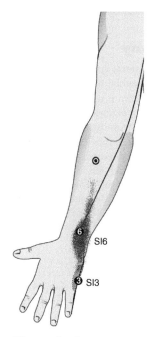

Effective distal points

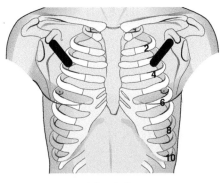

NL anterior

Motor function innervation: Radial nerve, C6, C7, C8
Nutrients: Ca, Mg, Fe, vit. B5, PUFA, phosphatase

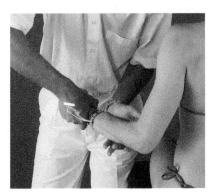

Extensor carpi ulnaris test

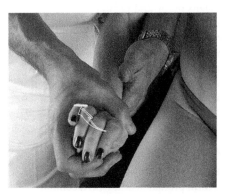

Extensor carpi ulnaris test, alternative view

Anatomy

Origin: Lateral epicondyle of the humerus and antebrachial fascia.

Course: From proximal to distal, lying between the extensor carpi ulnaris and the extensor carpi radialis.

Insertion: The four tendons radiate into the dorsal aponeurosis of the 2nd to the 5th fingers. Each tendon divides over the proximal phalanges into a middle tendon, which inserts at the base of the middle phalanx, and two lateral tendons, which insert at the base of the terminal phalanx.

Action

Together with the dorsal interossei it extends the proximal phalanges, as well as the middle and terminal phalanges, of the 2nd to 5th fingers. Helps in the extension of the wrist.

Signs of weakness: Extension in the proximal phalanx is difficult or restricted and an increased flexion of the wrist may be visible at rest.

Test

Position: The patient extends the wrist. The 2nd to 5th fingers are extended, or, according to Leaf (1996), the proximal phalanges are extended while the middle and terminal phalanges remain flexed.

Stabilization: The palmar aspect of the patient's hand in the area of the wrist.

Test contact: To the head of the proximal phalanx of the 2nd to 5th fingers.

Patient: Keeps the fingers at the proximal phalanges in extension.

Examiner: Resists attempting to flex the proximal phalanges.

Test errors, precautions: Over-powering the muscle during the test. Pressure must be administered precisely and with great sensitivity.

Myofascial syndrome

Stretch test: Extension at the elbow, forearm pronation and with a combined flexion of the wrist and all the joints of the fingers so that the fingertips are touching the palm of the hand.

PIR: From the stretch position the patient is asked to slowly extend the fingers of the metacarpophalangeal joints against the gentle resistance of the examiner. In the relaxation phase, the examiner gently elongates the muscle by returning the fingers to the stretch position.

Frequently found associated disorders

The muscle should always be tested when a compression syndrome of the radial nerve is suspected.

Compression weakness: Lesions of the root C7 from the C6/7 disc. Supinator (deep branch of the radial nerve), scalenus, costoclavicular and pectoralis minor syndromes.

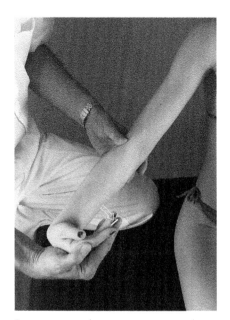

Post isometric relaxation: contraction phase

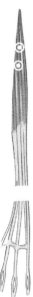

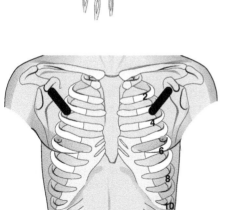

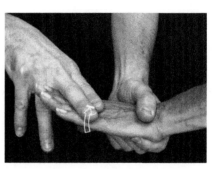

Effective distal point

NL

Motor function innervation:
Radial nerve, C6, C7, C8

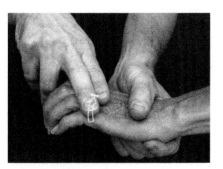

Extensor digitorum test

Alternative test of the extensor digitorum

Anatomy

Origin: Lateral tibial condyle, upper three-quarters of the fibula and the interosseous membrane.

Course: From a superior origin to an inferior insertion passing anterior and medially to the peroneus longus and brevis and deeper than and lateral to the tibialis anterior.

Insertion: Middle and terminal phalanx of the 2nd to 5th toes.

Action

Via the middle and terminal phalanges, extension of the 2nd to 5th toes, along with dorsal extension and pronation (eversion) of the foot. Plays a role in lateral stabilization of the ankle.

In synergy with the tibialis anterior it provides a breaking action, stopping the forefoot from a sudden foot drop following the heel strike. It also aids in holding the foot up in extension during the swing phase (Travell and Simons 1992). In individuals where the peroneus tertius muscle is absent, it takes over the function of lateral forefoot extension. Some even regard the peroneus tertius as a part of the extensor digitorum (Frick et al. 1992a, Frick et al. 1992b).

Signs of weakness: Hammertoes and excessive inversion foot when walking.

Test

Position: The foot of the patient is placed midway between plantar flexion and extension.

Stabilization: Cupping the hand under the area of the heel.

Test contact: To the head of the middle phalanx of the 2nd to 5th toes.

Patient: Extends the toes.

Examiner: Resists trying to flex the toes.

Test errors, precautions: The test position and the resistance directions must be precisely maintained. No pain should be caused by any of the hands doing the testing or stabilizing.

Myofascial syndrome

Stretch test: With the foot plantar flexed and inverted, the 2nd to 5th toes are maximally flexed.

PIR: Starting with the foot in the stretch position, the patient holds an inspiration for 7–10 s while slowly extending the toes. For the relaxation phase, the patient breathes out while the examiner brings the foot gently back to the stretch position to elongate the muscle.

Frequently found associated disorders

Lateral ankle instability, lateral shift lesions of the cuboids and tibiofibular syndesmosis lesions. Concomitant functional weakness of the peroneus tertius is a regular sequel to extensor digitorum longus weakness.

Compression weakness: Lesions of the root at L5 (disc L 4/5), iliolumbar ligament, piriformis and peroneus tunnel syndromes.

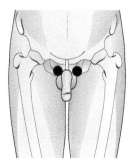
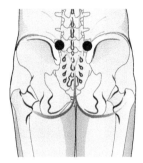
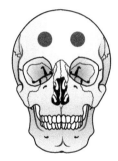

NL anterior   NL posterior   NV

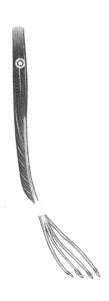

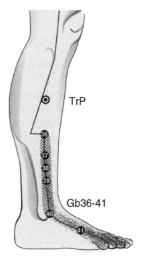

Effective distal points

Motor function innervation: Deep fibular nerve, L4, L5, S1
Rib pump: Intercostal space, costotransverse joint 3, 4, 8, 9
Organ: Bladder
Nutrients: Vitamin A, vitamin B complex with emphasis on B1 components, potassium
SRS: L1, L3, S3

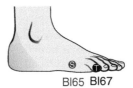

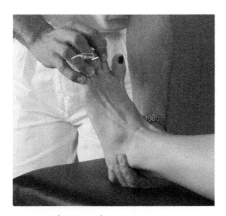

Extensor digitorum longus test

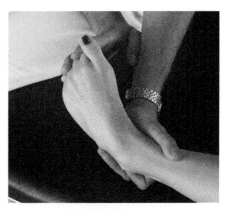

Post isometric relaxation

Anatomy

Origin: Distal part of the dorsal, lateral surface of the calcaneus.

Course: Diagonally from lateral to distal and medially over the foot below the tendons of the extensor digitorum longus.

Insertion: On the dorsal surface of the base of the proximal phalanx of the big toe.

Action

Extends the proximal phalanx of the big toe.

Signs of weakness: An increased flexion of the big toe.

Test

Position: The big toe is put into extension.

Stabilization: Primarily at the underside of the patient's 1st metatarsal bone.

Test contact: To the dorsal aspect of the head of the proximal phalanx of the big toe

Patient: Extends the big toe.

Examiner: Resists extension by flexing the big toe.

Test errors, precautions: Isolating the extensor hallucis brevis from the extensor hallucis longus is very difficult.

Myofascial syndrome

Stretch test: The foot is held in dorsiflexion (extension) to aid in isolating the brevis from the extensor hallucis longus and the proximal phalanx of the big toe is placed in maximum flexion.

PIR: The examiner contacts the proximal phalanx of the big toe and starting from the stretch position, provides gentle resistance while the patient slowly extends the toe. In the relaxation phase the big toe is brought back to the start position and slightly beyond.

Frequently found associated disorders

Compression weakness: Adverse tension in the peroneus longus and/or the extensor digitorum longus can affect the superficial and deep branches of the fibular nerve supply to the muscle.

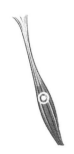

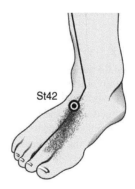

Trigger point and referred pain

Motor function innervation:
Deep fibular nerve: L5, S1
Spondylogenic reflex: L3

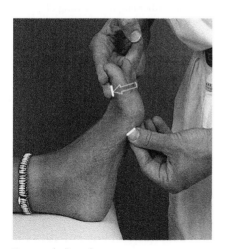

Extensor hallucis brevis test

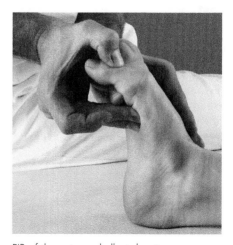

PIR of the extensor hallucis brevis

Anatomy

Origin: Middle three-quarters of the anterior surface of the fibula and interosseous membrane.

Course: Lying deep to the tibialis anterior, it progresses from superior to inferior.

Insertion: Base of the proximal phalanx of the big toe

Action

Extends the proximal phalanx and the terminal phalanx of the big toe. Supports dorsiflexion (extension) and supination of the foot.

Signs of weakness: An increased flexion of the terminal phalanx of the big toe.

Test

Position: Extension of the proximal phalanx of the big toe.

Stabilization: On the plantar aspect of the proximal phalanx.

Test contact: On the dorsum of the terminal phalanx.

Patient: Extends the big toe.

Examiner: Resists by attempting to flex the big toe at the distal phalanx.

Test errors, precautions: Poor fixation of the proximal phalanx of the big toe. This is more important than might be at first thought. Should the stabilization be insufficient, position changes of the proximal phalanx can produce false findings.

Myofascial syndrome

Stretch test: Full plantar flexion and inversion of the foot, with maximum flexion of all the joints of the big toe.

PIR: From the stretch position the patient is asked to extend the big toe against a gentle resistance by the examiner. In the relaxation phase the great toe is brought back to the stretch position and a bit more for a further slight stretching of the muscle.

Frequently found associated disorders

Compression weakness: For entrapment at the head of the fibula, see extensor hallucis brevis. Lesions of the L5 root from the L4/5 disc can lead to weakness of the muscle (Patten 1998, Walther 2000).

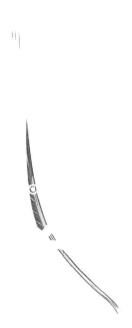

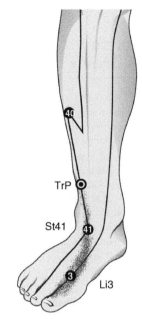

Trigger points and referred pain

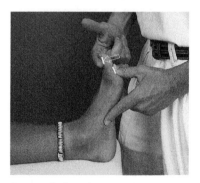

Extensor hallucis longus test

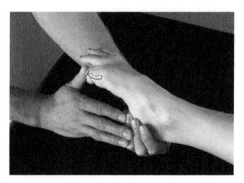

Post-isometric relaxation (PIR)

Motor function innervation: Deep fibular nerve, L5, S1
Spondylogenic reflex: L2

M. extensor pollicis brevis

Anatomy

Origin: The interosseous membrane, dorsal surface of the radius and distal to the origin of the abductor pollicis longus.

Course: The tendon runs over the styloid process of the radius and lies radial (lateral) to the extensor pollicis longus tendon. The muscle may be absent in some individuals and the tendon may even blend with that of the extensor longus.

Insertion: Dorsal surface of the proximal phalanx of the thumb.

Action

Primarily extends the proximal phalanx of the thumb, but helps with extension and abduction in the carpometacarpal joint and radial abduction in the wrist as well. Strangely, despite an apparent conflict in naming, its action is similar to that of the abductor pollicis longus, but because it involves the more distal joint, the terminology changes. (Note: With the hand in the anatomical position with the palm facing anterior, extension means that the thumb moves laterally away from the radial edge of the palm.)

Signs of weakness: Reduced strength in extending the proximal phalanx of the thumb and a possible increased flexion position at rest.

Test

Position: All the joints of the thumb are placed into extension.

Stabilization: With a broad contact to the palmar aspect of the hand and thumb. Special attention is made in fixating the metacarpophalangeal joint in extension.

Test contact: Over the dorsal surface of the proximal phalanx of the thumb.

Patient: Pulls the thumb into extension.

Examiner: Resists by gently pushing into flexion.

Test errors, precautions: Poor stabilization of the thumb and painful contact over the joints.

Frequently found associated disorders

The tendons of the abductor pollicis long. and brev. (anatomical 'snuff box') are a common site for tendosynovitis, especially in women between 30 and 50 years of age. This may lead to stenosing tenosynovitis (DeQuervain's disease).

Compression weakness: Entrapment of the radial nerve (thoracic inlet, radial nerve sulcus, supinator syndrome). Root lesions at C7 (intervertebral foramen C5/6).

M. extensor pollicis longus

Anatomy

Origin: Middle third of the dorsal surface of the ulna, interosseous membrane.

Course: From ulnar to radial and superior to inferior. Thereafter, the tendon runs within a small sulcus, over the distal end of the radius. With abduction and extension of the thumb, whereby the tendon of the extensor pollicis longus and abductor pollicis longus are visible, this is the tendon closest to the ulna.

Insertion: At the dorsal surface of the base of the distal phalanx of the thumb.

Action

Extends the distal phalanx of the thumb, helps with extension in the metacarpophalangeal joint and the proximal phalanx of the thumb. It also aids in radial abduction and extension in the wrist.

Note: With the hand in the anatomical position with respect to the rest of the body so that the palm is anterior, extension means that the thumb moves laterally away from the radial edge of the palm.

Signs of weakness: Increased flexion of the terminal phalanx of the thumb at rest.

Test

Position: All joints of the thumb are put into extension.

Stabilization: Broadly over the palmar aspect of the hand and thumb with special attention made in keeping both of the more proximal joints (metacarpophalangeal and 1st interphalangeal) in extension.

Test contact: On the dorsal surface of the terminal phalanx of the thumb.

Patient: Extends the terminal phalanx of the thumb.

Examiner: Resists by carefully pushing the terminal phalanx into flexion.

Test errors, precautions: Poor stabilization of the thumb in extension and pain caused by the contact in the area of the thumbnail.

Frequently found associated disorders

Tenosynovitis around Lister's tubercle especially following fracture of the radius or Colles fracture of both the radius and ulnar bones (skier's thumb).

Compression weakness: Entrapment of the radial nerve leading to extension weakness of the terminal phalanx of the thumb. Weakness may be compensated by contraction of the abductor pollicis and the transverse fibres of the adductor pollicis brevis muscles that are innervated by the median and ulnar nerves, respectively. Both muscles radiate into the dorsal aponeurosis of the hand and may adversely influence the interossei and lumbricales.

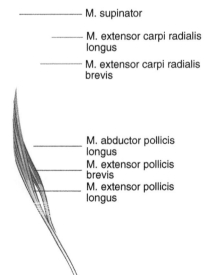

———————— M. supinator

———— M. extensor carpi radialis longus

———— M. extensor carpi radialis brevis

———— M. abductor pollicis longus

———— M. extensor pollicis brevis

———— M. extensor pollicis longus

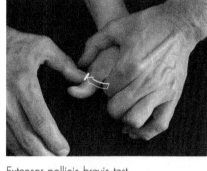

Extensor pollicis brevis test

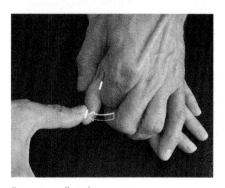

Extensor pollicis longus test

Motor function innervation:
Deep branch of the radial nerve, C6, C7, C8

M. flexor carpi radialis

Anatomy

Origin: Medial epicondyle of the humerus and the antebrachial fascia covering the flexor digitorum superficialis lying deep to the flexor carpi radialis.

Course: Proximally it passes down the forearm medial to the pronator teres and lateral to the palmaris longus. Distally, in the superficial muscle layer, its tendon is flanked by the brachioradialis radially and the palmaris longus on the ulnar side.

Insertion: On the surface of the palm at the base of the 2nd metacarpal bone and with a few fibres at the base of the 3rd metacarpal.

Action

Flexion and radial abduction of the hand. Helps in pronation and flexion of the elbow joint.

Signs of weakness: In a few cases, an increased ulnar adduction of the hand may be seen and, more rarely, increased wrist extension. More often, indications of weakness will be noted with use rather than in a static position.

Test

Position: The forearm is externally rotated to a position of about 75% of full supination. Thereafter the wrist is flexed and radially abducted.

Stabilization: Supporting underneath, on the dorsum of the patient's distal forearm, close to the wrist.

Test contact: At the ball of the thumb as distally as is possible without causing discomfort or pain.

Patient: Flexes and radial abducts the wrist.

Examiner: Resists by pressing the hand into extension and slight ulnar adduction.

Test errors, precautions: Poor fixation of the forearm and wrist. Any elbow flexion during the test will activate the biceps, change the resistance angle, weaken the stabilization, shorten all synergistic wrist flexors and probably falsify the findings.

Myofascial syndrome

Stretch test

The elbow is supported from below and fully extended, followed by ulnar adduction and extension of the wrist.

PIR

From the stretch position, the patient slowly flexes the wrist toward the radial side. In the relaxation phase, the examiner gently elongates the muscle by bringing the hand back to the stretch position.

Frequently found associated disorders

Compression weakness

Root lesions involving C7 from the C6/C7 intervertebral foramen, thoracic inlet and pronator teres syndrome.

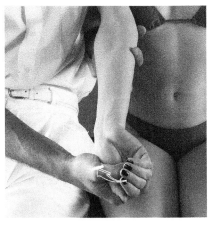

Post isometric relaxation

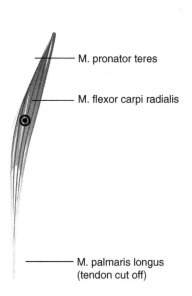

M. pronator teres

M. flexor carpi radialis

M. palmaris longus
(tendon cut off)

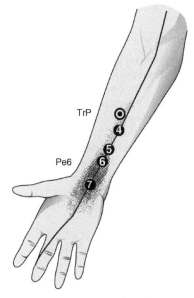

TrP

Pe6

Trigger points and referred pain

Motor function innervation:
Median nerve, C6, C7, C8

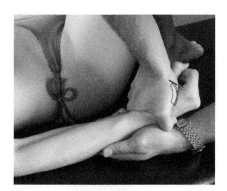

Flexor carpi radialis test

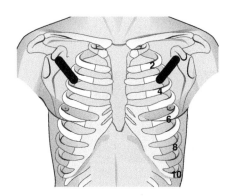

NL anterior

M. flexor carpi ulnaris

Anatomy

Origin: Humeral head: From the common flexor tendon on the ulnar (medial) epicondyle of the humerus.

Ulnar head: Medial part of the olecranon, proximal two-thirds of the ulna and antebrachial fascia.

Course: Between the ulnar margin and the flexor digitorum superficialis.

Insertion: Directly onto the pisiform and, indirectly, through ligamentous attachments, to the hamate and base of the 5th metacarpal bones.

Action: Flexion and ulnar adduction of the wrist and supports elbow flexion.

Signs of weakness: Infrequently, radial abduction may be apparent, but reduced strength when bending the wrist is a more common finding.

Test

Position: The forearm is put into full supination followed by the patient flexing the wrist to the ulnar side.

Stabilization: Underneath, on the dorsum of the patient's distal forearm, close to the wrist.

Test contact: On the palmar, ulnar aspect of the hand, over the ball of the little finger.

Patient: Flexes the wrist, keeping it in ulnar adduction.

Examiner: Resists pushing the ulnar side of the hand into extension and slight radial abduction.

Test errors, precautions: As with the flexor carpi radialis, poor fixation of the forearm and wrist. Any elbow flexion during the test will activate the biceps, change the resistance angle, weaken the stabilization, shorten all synergistic wrist flexors and probably falsify any finding.

Myofascial syndrome

Stretch test: The elbow is supported from below and extended; followed by radial abduction and extension of the hand.

PIR: From the stretch position the patient slowly contracts the muscle to flex the wrist to the ulnar side. In the relaxation phase, a gentle elongation of the muscle is made by the examiner returning the hand to the stretch position.

Frequently found associated disorders

Symptoms similar to those found in 'epicondylopathia' ulnaris humeri or 'golfer's elbow'.

Compression weakness: Root lesions of C8 from the C7/C8 intervertebral foramen, thoracic inlet and sulcus ulnaris syndrome.

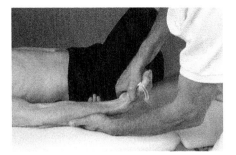

Group test of flexor carpi radialis and ulnaris. The hand is flexed without radial abduction or ulnar adduction

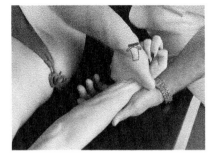

Flexor carpi ulnaris test

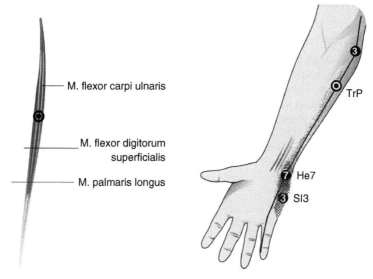

M. flexor carpi ulnaris

M. flexor digitorum superficialis

M. palmaris longus

TrP

He7

SI3

Trigger points and referred pain

Motor function innervation:
Ulnar nerve, C7, C8, T1

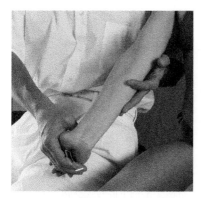

Elongation and PIR: contraction phase

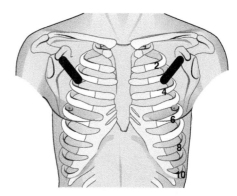

NL anterior

M. flexor digiti minimi

Anatomy

Origin: From the hamulus portion of the hamate bone and the flexor retinaculum on the palmar side of the hand.

Course: Superficial to the opponens digiti minimi and on a plane parallel with the abductor digiti minimi.

Insertion: At the base of the proximal phalanx of the little finger.

Action

Flexes the proximal phalanx of the little finger and aids in opposition of the little finger.

Signs of weakness: A poor opposition position of the little finger noted by difficulty in arriving at the halfway point when attempting to cross the palm.

Test

Position: All the distal joints of the little finger are kept straight, in extension, and flexion is made only at the proximal phalanx.

Stabilization: Grasping the 5th metacarpal mainly on the dorsum, but also over the palmar side of the hand.

Test contact: To the head of the proximal phalanx of the little finger. Alternatively, the testing finger may make contact over the entire palmar surface of the little finger. This will aid in keeping the distal joints in extension.

Patient: Keeping the finger straight, flexes the little finger.

Examiner: Resists by pulling the little finger into extension.

Test errors, precautions: It is easy to utilize too much strength during the test. The most common error is when resistance is made in a 'bottle opener' fashion by keeping the hand fixed and using the entire forearm as a lever against the little finger.

Myofascial syndrome

Stretch test: A slightly exaggerated hyper-extension of the little finger will provoke referred pain if a myofascial problem is present.

PIR: Starting from the stretch position, the patient slowly flexes the little finger against minimal resistance by the examiner. A gradual extension is performed in the relaxation phase to return the finger to the stretch position and, then, slightly beyond.

Frequently found associated disorders

Compression syndrome of the ulnar nerve in the wrist, especially from the pisiform-hamate area. The muscle can also be used as the indicator from disc lesions found at C7/T1 (nerve root C8).

Compression weakness: Thoracic inlet, sulcus ulnaris, ulnar tunnel and pisiform-hamate syndromes.

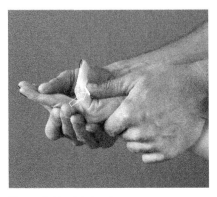

Flexor digiti minimi test

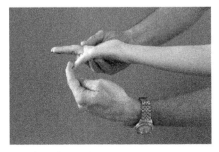

PIR of M. flexor digiti minimi: contraction phase

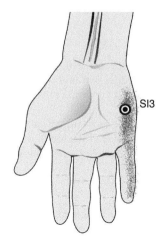

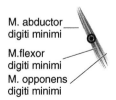

M. abductor
digiti minimi

M.flexor
digiti minimi

M. opponens
digiti minimi

Trigger points and referred pain

Motor function innervation: Ulnar nerve, C8, T1

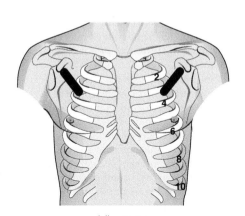

NL anterior

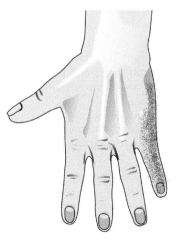

Trigger points and referred pain

Anatomy

Origin: Medial process of the calcaneal tuberosity, middle part of the plantar aponeurosis and bordering intermuscular septa.

Course: It is the most superficial of the muscles of the sole of the foot.

Insertion: At the middle phalanges of the 2nd to 5th toes.

Action

Flexes the middle phalanges of 2nd to 5th toes and helps with flexion of the proximal phalanges.

Signs of weakness: Lack of support for the arch of the foot so that a 'flexible arch' will be noted, where the arch tends to droop and flatten out when bearing weight, but returns to a more normal position when not.

Test

Position: Flexion of the toes.

Stabilization: In a broad fashion on the dorsum of the foot covering the metatarsals.

Test contact: To the plantar surface of the middle phalanx of the 2nd to 5th toes.

Patient: Flexes the toes as much as possible.

Examiner: Resists trying to 'peel' the toes into extension.

When there is normal strength of the flexor digitorum brevis and longus the middle phalanges will flex along with the terminal phalanges. However, if the flexor digitorum longus is weak, the terminal phalanges will remain extended and only the middle phalanges will flex.

Test errors, precautions: Difficulty in differentiation from the m. flexor digitorum longus.

Myofascial syndrome

Stretch test: The foot is kept in a neutral position, the plantar aspect of the terminal phalanges are held and the toes are maximally extended by pulling and holding them in dorsal extension.

PIR: Starting from the stretch position the patient is asked to slowly flex the toes against the examiner's resistance. In the relaxation phase the toes are brought back to the stretch position and slightly beyond.

Frequently found associated disorders

Any shortening of the gastrocnemius or soleus muscles or the Achilles tendon may lead to 'plantar fasciitis'. Increased tension of the plantar aponeurosis is frequently associated with trigger points in the area of the intrinsic plantar foot muscles. Shoes with inflexible soles that restrict movement of the toes can also cause the condition.

Compression weakness: Root lesions of S1 from the L5/S1 intervertebral foramen, iliolumbar ligament and piriformis syndrome.

Tarsal tunnel syndrome where the posterior tibial nerve is entrapped as it passes through the tunnel posterior to the medial malleolus. Fallen arches, anteroflexion of the calcaneous bone, injuries to the ankle mortise and space occupying lesions, can all compress the nerve. In a few cases compression of the tibial nerve in the area of the tendinous arch of the soleus can also occur.

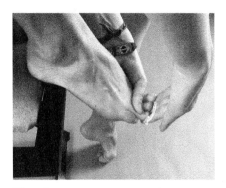

PIR, self-treatment: contraction phase

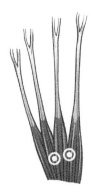

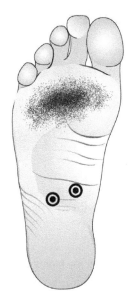

Trigger points and referred pain

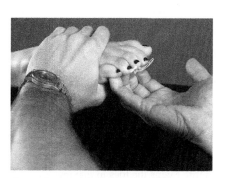

Motor function innervation:
Medial plantar nerve (L5), S1
Nutrients: Phosphatase for
tarsal tunnel syndrome

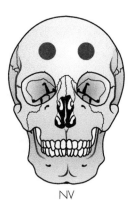

Flexor digitorum brevis test

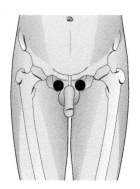

NL anterior

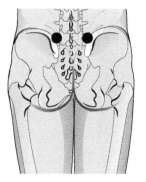

NL posterior

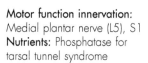

NV

Anatomy

Origin: On the posterior fascia of the tibia, distal to the origin of the soleus.

Course: Deep to the soleus, follows the tibia distally.

Insertion: At the base of the terminal phalanges of the 2nd to 5th toes.

Action

Flexes the terminal phalanges of the 2nd to 5th toes and helps with flexion of the proximal phalanges.

Aids in medial stabilization of the foot as well as the longitudinal arch. The effect is enhanced when the foot is in plantar flexion and inversion.

During gait it is active throughout the entire stance phase until push off. When standing it also helps in maintaining and fine-tuning static balance.

Signs of weakness: Lack of support for the arch of the foot, plantar pain during or following long walking or standing on the toes.

Test

Position: Flexed toes.

Stabilization: Middle phalanx of the 2nd to 5th toes.

Test contact: To the terminal phalanges of the toes.

Patient: Keeps the toes in maximal flexion.

Examiner: Resists by attempting to 'peel' the toes into extension.

Test errors, precautions: Differentiation between it and the flexor digitorum brevis may be difficult. Cramping of the plantar muscles during testing is common.

Myofascial syndrome

Stretch test: The foot is dorsiflexed (extended) and everted (pronation). The plantar aspect of the terminal phalanges of the toes are contacted and pulled into full extension.

PIR: From the stretch position the patient is asked to flex the toes against a modest resistance by the examiner. In the relaxation phase the examiner gently elongates the muscle by returning the toes to the stretch position and slightly beyond.

Frequently found associated disorders

The development of hammer toes especially noted in chronic tarsal tunnel syndrome where the flexor digitorum longus function remains intact but the flexor digitorum is weak.

Compression weakness: Root lesions of S1 from the L5/S1 intervertebral foramen, iliolumbar ligament and piriformis syndrome.

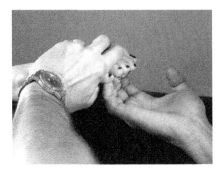

Flexor digitorum brevis test

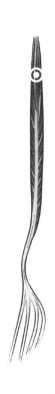

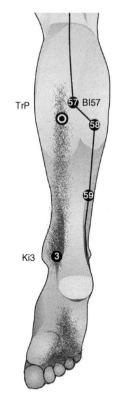

Trigger points and referred pain

Motor function innervation: Tibial nerve, L5, S1
Nutrients: Phosphatase for tarsal tunnel syndrome
SRS: L3, L4, L5

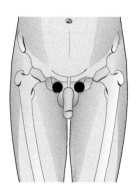

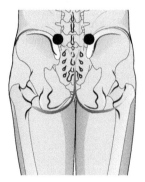

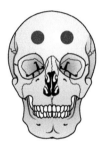

NL anterior   NL posterior   NV

Anatomy

Origin: On an area covering about 75% of the proximal anteromedial surface of the ulna, interosseous membrane and antebrachial fascia.

Course: Lies in the third layer of the volar (anterior) muscles of the forearm. The distal tendons of the muscle run through a passage made up of the tendons of the flexor digitorum superficialis.

Insertion: Divided into four individual tendons at the base of the terminal phalanges of the 2nd to 5th fingers.

Action

Flexes the terminal phalanges of the 2nd to 5th fingers and, aids in the flexion of the middle and proximal phalanges. To some extent it is also associated with wrist flexion.

Signs of weakness: It is the only muscle that flexes the most distal phalanges. Weakness is especially apparent when attempting to grasp small objects.

Test

Position: The proximal and middle phalanges of the finger are kept in extension and the distal phalanx is flexed.

Stabilization: The examiner grasps the patient's hand so that both proximal phalanges are kept in extension, allowing only flexion at the most distal joint.

Test contact: At the flexed, terminal phalanx.

Patient: Flexes only the terminal phalanx of the finger.

Examiner: Using only the thumb and index fingers, attempts to extend the distal phalanx.

Test errors, precautions: Care must be taken not to use a 'bottle opener' approach whereby the thumb and index fingers remain fixed and the resistance pressure is applied by the arm and shoulder. No pain should be caused during stabilization and the force of the testing resistance should be adjusted according to patient's age and capacity.

Myofascial syndrome

Stretch test: This test can only be made together with the flexor digitorum superficialis. The elbow is slightly flexed to take the wrist flexors out of the test. The wrist and fingers are then maximally extended.

PIR: From the stretch position, the patient slowly flexes the fingers. The examiner gently elongates the muscle by bringing the fingers back to the stretch position for the relaxation phase.

Cause for compression: According to Travell and Simons (1983) increased tension in the flexor digitorum superficiales and profundus may compress the ulnar nerve as it progresses from the elbow into the forearm and hand.

Frequently found associated disorders

Compression syndromes: Cervical lesions of the 8th root from the C7/Th1 IVF and disc. Peripheral nerve compression of the thoracic outlet, sulcus ulnaris (ulnar nerve, 4th and 5th fingers) and pronator teres (median nerve, 2nd and 3rd fingers) syndromes, are all common findings.

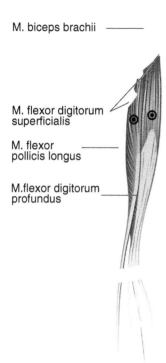

M. biceps brachii

M. flexor digitorum superficialis

M. flexor pollicis longus

M.flexor digitorum profundus

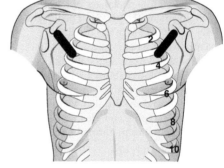

TrP

TrP

Pe6

He7

SI3

Trigger points and referred pain

Motor function innervation:
2nd and 3rd finger:
Median nerve, C7, C8, T1
4th and 5th finger:
Ulnar nerve, C7, C8, T1

NL anterior

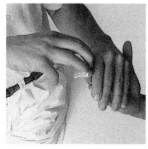

A general test of the left flexor digitorum profundus (e.g. for entrapments proximal to the elbow)

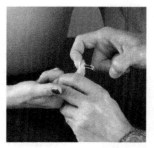

Individual testing of the right deep flexor digitorum (e.g. for entrapments in or after the cubital tunnel)

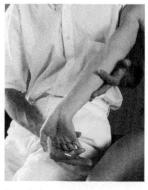

Stretch test and PIR

Anatomy

Origin: Humeral head: Medial epicondyle of the humerus, ulnar collateral ligament and the antebrachial fascia.

Ulnar head: Medial side of the coronoid process of the ulna.

Radial head: From the anterior surface of the radius, arising from below the pronator teres muscle.

Course: Lies in the 2nd layer of the volar (anterior) forearm. It is sandwiched over a wide area between the deeper flexor digitorum profundus and flexor pollicis longus muscles (3rd layer) and the more superficial brachioradialis, flexor carpi radialis and palmaris longus muscles.

Insertion: With four individual tendons on both sides of the middle phalanges of the 2nd to 5th fingers.

Action

Flexes the middle phalanges of the 2nd to 5th fingers on the proximal phalanges. Helps in the flexion of the proximal phalanges and wrist.

Signs of weakness: Difficulty in making a fist and a reduced ability to use the fingers when the proximal finger joints are in extension and the distal joints in flexion. For example, typing and playing the piano would be activities performed with some difficulty.

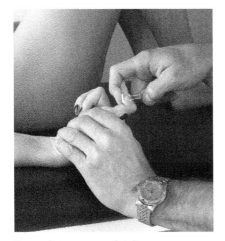

Flexor digitorum superficialis test

Test

Position: The hand of the patient is supinated and the proximal phalanx of the finger to be tested is kept in extension.

Stabilization: The dorsum of the hand is held in supination and the most proximal phalanges of the hands and fingers are kept in extension.

Patient: Bends the proximal interphalangeal joint.

Test contact: The distal-most joint of the finger is kept in extension in a pincer-like fashion grasping the distal phalanges between the thumb and forefinger. This helps to maintain control of the finger during the actual test.

Examiner: Attempts to extend the fingers at the middle phalanx.

Test errors, precautions: Insufficient or improper stabilization of the hand and the proximal phalanges.

Pain in the finger joints during test might compromise the test and should be avoided if possible.

Myofascial syndrome

Stretch test: The elbow is slightly flexed to keep the wrist flexors out of the test and the terminal phalanges are allowed to slightly and naturally flex to keep the flexor digitorum profundus out of the test. This is followed by grasping the middle phalanges to keep the proximal interphalangeal joint in extension.

PIR: From the stretched position, the patient slowly flexes the middle phalanx to contract the muscles. In the relaxation phase the finger is gently brought back to the stretch position by the examiner.

Possible causes for nerve compression: Ulnar nerve entrapment may be caused by compressive forces from the proximal part of the flexor digitorum superficialis.

Frequently found associated disorders

This muscle can aid in the differential diagnosis of peripheral entrapment syndromes of the median nerve originating prior to the carpal tunnel at the wrist.

Compression weakness: It is a good muscle for evaluation of C8 root irritation from the intervertebral foramen lesions of C7/C8 and peripheral entrapment of the median nerve by the pronator teres.

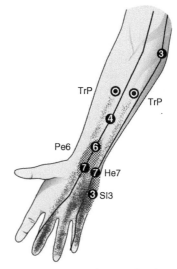

Trigger points and pain referral

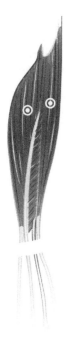

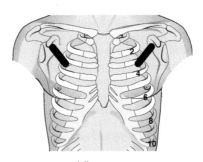

NL anterior

Motor function innervation:
Median nerve, C7, C8, T1

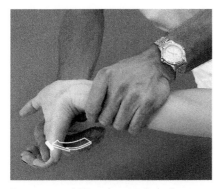

Extension and PIR with extended elbow

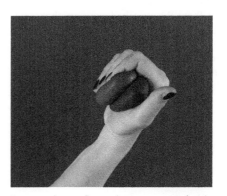

Training the m. flexor digitorium superficialis

Anatomy

Origin: 1st to 3rd cuneiform bones, the plantar calcaneocuboid ligament and posterior tibial tendon.

Course: From posterior to anterior in the superficial layer of the plantar muscles.

Insertion: Medial and lateral sides of the base of the proximal phalanx of the big toe.

Action

Flexes the proximal phalanx of the big toe.

Signs of weakness: Hammer toe and reduced stability of the longitudinal arch of the foot.

Test

Position: Great toe is flexed at the metatarsophalangeal joint.

Stabilization: The forefoot and, in particular, the 1st metatarsal bone.

Test contact: With the fingers on the plantar aspect of the proximal phalanx of the great toe. The thumb may stabilize the dorsal aspect of the toe.

Patient: Flexes the great toe.

Examiner: Pulls on the proximal phalanx attempting to bring the great toe into extension at the metatarsophalangeal joint.

Myofascial syndrome

Stretch test: The big toe is put into maximal extension with the foot held in plantar flexion (to take the flexor hallucis longus out of the test). When the test is positive, referred pain and cramping of the muscle may be provoked.

PIR: From the stretched position, the patient is asked to flex the big toe while the examiner gently resists the movement. The toe is then brought slowly back into extension by the examiner during the relaxation phase.

Frequently found associated disorders

Weakness of the muscle occurs with tarsal tunnel syndrome. Often, weakness of the muscle is not immediately noted and can be 'hidden' during normal testing. Only when the foot is place in certain positions of increased mechanical stress will the weakness become apparent. For example, weakness may become evident only when standing. One of the probable causes of this is from a breakdown in medial ankle stability due to dysfunction of the tibialis posterior muscle. Classically, pain will be experienced in the forefoot after walking. As a consequence, trigger points develop in the deep intrinsic muscles of the foot; especially in the flexor hallucis brevis. As well, it is often accompanied by numbness, swelling and cramping of the plantar aspect of the foot. Any malfunction in the biomechanics of the foot can lead to ascending disorders. This is understood to mean that the foot will cause structural problems above it and ultimately involve the knee, hips, pelvis, the spine, neck and TMJ.

Compression related weaknesses: Tarsal tunnel syndrome, piriformis syndrome, S1 root lesion (disc L5/S1).

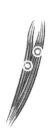

Trigger points and referred pain pattern.

Motor function innervation: Medial plantar nerve (L5), S1, S2, S3
Nutrients: Phosphatase for tarsal tunnel syndrome
SRS: L1

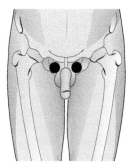

Test of flexor hallucis brevis

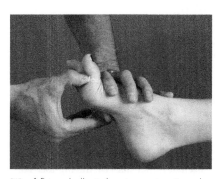

PIR of flexor hallucis brevis: contraction phase

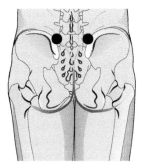

NL anterior

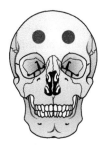

NL posterior

NV

Anatomy

Origin: Posterior surface of the distal two-thirds of the fibula, interosseous membrane and posterior intermuscular septum.

Course: Together with the flexor digitorum longus, they form the deepest muscle layer of the posterior lower leg. The tendon runs parallel to the flexor digitorum longus, the tibialis posterior, the tibial nerve and the posterior tibial artery and vein. Together they pass through the tarsal tunnel; it's borders formed by the calcaneus and talus bones on the lateral (deep) aspect and medially (superficially) by the retinaculum flexorum ligament.

Insertion: Base of the terminal phalanx of the big toe.

Action

Flexes the terminal phalanx at the interphalangeal joint of the big toe and will assist the flexor hallicis brevis in flexing the metatarsophalangeal joint. Aids in plantar flexion and inversion of the foot, especially when the toe is in extension.

Signs of weakness: Disorders are seen during gait, primarily. The muscle may be weak when push off is seen to be made more laterally by the 3rd and 4th digits of the forefoot rather than by the big toe. This is due to an outward rolling of the foot, in part, caused by a weakness of this muscle and/or the peroneus longus.

Test

Position: The patient's foot is perpendicular to the table and the big toe is slghtly extended.

Stabilization: Made on the forefoot and proximal phalanx. The interphalangeal joint of the big toe is kept in extension.

Test contact: On the plantar aspect of the terminal phalanx of the big toe. The terminal phalanx may be grabbed in a pincer fashion.

Patient: Flexes the big toe.

Examiner: Tries to extend the proximal phalanx of the big toe.

The test may also be done in a standing position in order to reveal hidden weaknesses, although this is obviously more difficult. Poor stabilization of the sustentaculum tali and medial arch of the foot by the posterior tibialis muscle is the usual cause. As a consequence, the tarsal tunnel is compromised and the tibial nerve entrapped.

Testing errors, precautions: Inadequate stabilization of the proximal phalanx and interphalangeal joint of the big toe, allowing it to flex as well. Excessive stabilization pressure by the examiner on the proximal phalanx of the big toe. The novice may tend to use a 'can-opener' move whereby the fingers and wrist are fixed and the resistance is made by the arm and shoulder muscles. The lever action is just too great for most patients to overcome.

Myofascial syndrome

Stretch test: The foot is put into dorsiflexion and eversion (pronation) and the great toe is fully extended. This position could activate trigger points in both the calf muscles and the flexor digitorum longus.

PIR: From the stretch position, the patient gently flexes the interphalangeal joints of the big toe while the examiner holds the metatarsophalangeal joint as well as the foot in dorsal extension. During the relaxation phase, the examiner slowly brings the joint back into extension.

Frequently found associated disorders

Tarsal tunnel syndrome, where the diagnostic indicator is that the flexor hallucis longus functions normally, but the flexor hallicus brevis is weak. The flexor hallucis brevis has an innervation distal to the tarsal tunnel and will be weaker than the flexor hallucis longus. A classic hammer toe anomaly will develop as the condition becomes chronic.

Compression weaknesses: S1 root lesion due to disc lesions or other foraminal bottlenecks. (Walther 2000), piriformis syndrome.

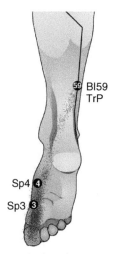

59 Bl59
TrP

Sp4 4

Sp3 3

Trigger point and referred pain pattern

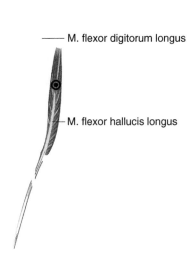

M. flexor digitorum longus

M. flexor hallucis longus

Motor function innervation:
Tibial nerve, L5, S1, S2
SRS: L3, L4

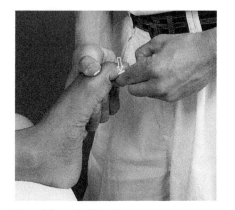

Test of flexor hallucis longus

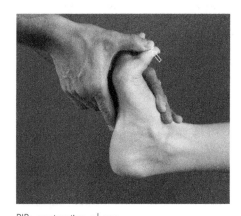

PIR: contraction phase

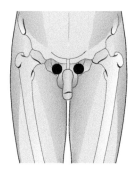

NL anterior

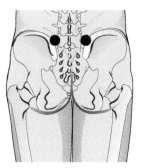

NL posterior

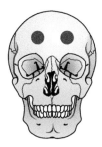

NV

Anatomy

Origin: Superficial head: Flexor retinaculum and trapezium bone.

Deep head: Trapezium and capitate bones.

Course: Lies parallel to the opponens pollicis.

Insertion: Radial side of the base of the proximal phalanx of the thumb.

Action

Flexes the proximal phalanx of the thumb. It flexes the 1st metacarpal bone and aids in the opposition of the thumb.

Signs of weakness: Difficulties holding a pen.

Test

Position: The thumb is adducted so that it's internal edge rests on the palmar edge of the hand, close to the index finger. Keeping the interphalangeal joint in extension, it is flexed at the metacarpophalangeal joint.

Stabilization: On the 1st metacarpal.

Test contact: Using the index finger and thumb in a pincer-like contact, the examiner grasps the ulnar and palmar aspect of the proximal phalanx of the thumb.

Patient: Flexes the metacarpophalangeal joint of the thumb so that it crosses over the palm towards the little finger.

Examiner: Pulls the proximal phalanx of the thumb away from the middle of the palm attempting to take it into extension.

Testing errors, precautions: A distinction is made between the flexor pollicis brevis and opponens pollicis by the test contact: For the opponens, the contact is to the head of the 1st metacarpal and the flexor pollicis brevis is tested close to the palm while the opponens pollicis is elevated from it.

Myofascial syndrome

Stretch test: The thumb is extended at both joints.

PIR: From the stretched position, the patient slowly flexes the thumb. The examiner gently elongates the muscle by returning the thumb to the stretch position in the relaxation phase.

Frequently found associated disorders

'Trigger thumb', whereby the thumb tends to become locked in flexion and only with external help is it possible to return the joint into extension. It is commonly associated with a trigger point in the flexor pollicis brevis that restricts movement of the flexor pollicis longus tendon.

Compression weaknesses: Compression disorders are not commonly found due to the dual innervation of the muscle by the median and ulnar nerves.

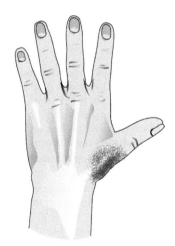

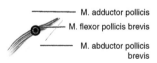

M. adductor pollicis
M. flexor pollicis brevis
M. abductor pollicis brevis

Motor function innervation:
Superficial head: Median nerve, C6, C7, C8, T1
Deep head: Ulnar nerve, C8, T1

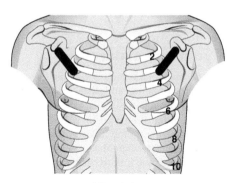

NL anterior

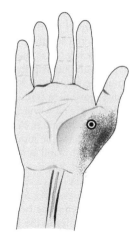

Trigger points and pain referral

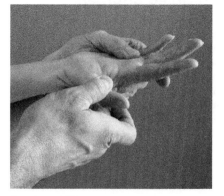

Stretch and PIR

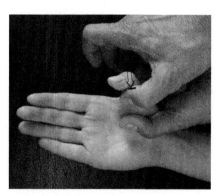

Flexor pollicis brevis test

M. flexor pollicis longus

Anatomy

Origin: Has multiple insertions and begins distal to the radial tuberosity on the anterior surface of the radius, the interosseous membrane and the medial margin of the coronoid process and/or the medial epicondyle of the humerus.

Course: Lies in the deep muscle layer of the forearm.

Insertion: At the palmar surface of the base of the terminal phalanx of the thumb.

Action

Flexes the interphalangeal joint of the thumb. Also aids in flexion of the metacarpophalangeal joints.

In this context, flexion means flexing the interphalangeal joint of the thumb on the thumb itself. Anatomically the thumb's position in space is related to the hand, not the body, and any description of movement must be made with respect to the hand. Thus, movement of the thumb from above the palm and towards the palm is considered adduction. When the thumb is resting close to the index finger, on the level of the palm and is moved to the centre of the hand, it is described as flexion. It is important not to confuse the movement, as it is imperative to understand when attempting to isolate and test the different muscles in the thumb. For the flexor pollicis longus, the examiner must resist only the flexion at the distal joint of the thumb on itself.

Signs of weakness: The ability to flex the terminal phalanx of the thumb is reduced. Difficulties in holding small objects like a pen.

Test

Position: The interphalangeal joint of the thumb is flexed and the metacarpophalangeal joint is held in extension.

Stabilization: With a firm grasp over the 1st metacarpal and proximal phalanx of the thumb to keep it in extension. If the thumb of the examiner is placed along the axis of the anterior thumb so that it ends just below the interphalangeal joint, it will tend to keep the flexion component restricted to that joint alone.

Testing contact: On the pad of terminal phalanx of the thumb or, using a pincer-like contact covering both the anterior and posterior aspects of the terminal phalanx.

Patient: Flexes the distal thumb while the examiner keeps the proximal joints of the thumb in extension.

Examiner: Attempts to extend the terminal phalanx of the thumb.

Test errors, precautions: Incorrect stabilization (allowing flexion of the first interphalangeal joint). Too much resistance-pressure by the examiner, causing pain.

Myofascial syndrome

Stretch test: The thumb is extended at both the proximal and distal interphalangeal joints.

PIR: From the stretch position, the patient gently flexes the thumb followed by the relaxation phase where the examiner gently extends the thumb back to the stretch position.

Frequently found associated disorders

The muscle is innervated by the median nerve, but proximal to the carpal tunnel. It is therefore useful in differential diagnosis of median nerve compression syndromes as well as C8 root syndrome (intervertebral foramen C7/T1). 'Trigger thumb' is also related to dysfunction of this muscle.

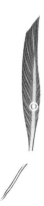

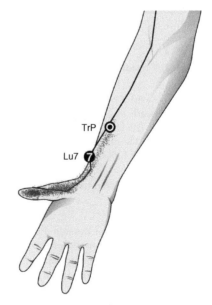

Trigger points and referred pain pattern

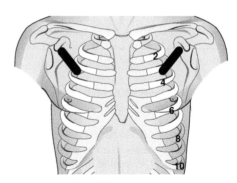

Motor function innervation:
Median nerve, C7, C8, T1

NL anterior

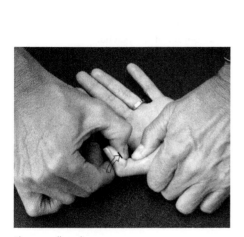

Flexor pollicis longus test

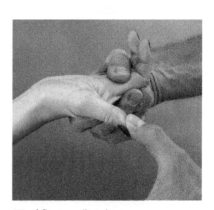

PIR of flexor pollicis longus

Anatomy

Origin: Medial head: Medial condyle of the femur.
Lateral head: Lateral condyle of the femur.
Course: Both heads attach to the broad Achilles tendon. The larger medial head is also longer and the muscle ends more distally towards the foot than the lateral head.
Insertion: At the calcaneal tuberosity.

Action

Primarily plantar flexion of the foot, but it also aids in flexion at the knee joint.
Signs of weakness: Hyperextension of the knee when standing and instability when walking on tiptoes.

Test

Classic test

Position: The test may be made with the patient lying either on his abdomen or on his back. The knee is kept in extension for both positions and the foot is plantar flexed.
Test contact: One hand firmly grasps the patient's heel and the other holds the forefoot.
Patient: Plantar flexes the forefoot.
Examiner: Attempts to push the forefoot into dorsiflexion (extension of the foot) while simultaneously pulling down (caudally) on the heel.

In this test, the gastrocnemius cannot be isolated from the soleus.

The above is the classic method of testing the gastrocnemius muscle according to Kendall and Kendall (1983), Walther (1981), and Leaf (1996). The test primarily evaluates plantar flexion capacity of the foot. While the test does tend to better isolate the muscle, due to the very short lever afforded to the examiner and the overall strength of the two muscles, even in a very weakened state, the test will show apparently normal strength. Only when massive weakness of the muscle is found, as seen in those having difficulty standing on the toes, does the test tend to be indicative. Otherwise, it is quite inadequate to the task, to say the least.

Beardall test (1985)

This test is more useful and evidences weakness patterns in the muscle more often than the one above. It is designed to primarily evaluate the flexion capacity at the knee joint rather than the plantar flexion of the foot. More importantly, a much longer lever is afforded in which to exert counter-pressure. The test is not without some drawbacks, however. Significant synergism is evolved from the strong hamstring and the gracilis muscles.
Position: The patient lies supine with the hips and knees flexed. The knee is flexed about 80–90° and the foot is flexed so that its plantar aspect is resting on the table surface as much as possible.
Stabilization: With a broad contact on the anterior aspect of the knee, close to the lower border of the patella.

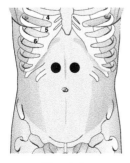

NL anterior

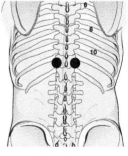

NL posterior

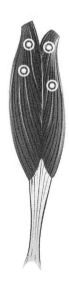
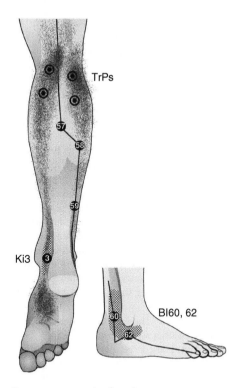

Trigger points and referred pain pattern

Motor function innervation: Tibial nerve, L4, L5, S1, S2
Rib pump: Intercostal space, costotransverse joint 6, 7
Meridian: Pericardium Circulation-Sex
Organ: Adrenal glands
Nutrients: Co-factors of adrenal enzymes: Vit. B2, B5, B6, B9, B12, C, tyrosine
SRS:
Medial head: L1 and L2
Lateral head: L2

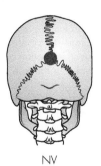

NV

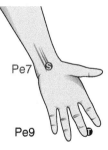

Test contact: The hand curls behind and firmly grasps the posterior part of the calcaneus. The forearm and elbow of the examiner should rest on the table surface. The contact should not be painful.

Patient: Draws the heel toward the buttocks by sliding it along the table surface. Important note: During the test the heel of the patient must **not** elevate from the table surface. Elevation brings the hamstrings into the test and may negate weakness.

Examiner: Attempts to extend the knee by pulling on the calcaneus. Important note: The best way to keep the resistance vector parallel to the table surface is for the examiner to keep the elbow and forearm on the surface of the table. Elevation of the elbow tends to change the resistance direction and bring the hamstring muscles into the test.

Lateral head: The examiner laterally rotates the tibia so that the foot points externally. The contact hand used should be internal to the leg of the patient, otherwise the forearm of the examiner will come to rest on the externally rotated forefoot. The arm will be automatically raised from the table and possibly negate weakness findings.

Medial head: The examiner rotates the tibia medially so that the foot points internally. The contact hand is changed and placed laterally for the same reasons as above. Direction of resistance for both individual heads is the same as for both together.

Test errors, precautions: Most importantly, the patient must neither lift the foot off the table nor push it more firmly on to the surface. In all cases of apparent weakness, the hamstrings must be tested. If the hamstrings and/or the synergistic flexors of the knee at the thigh are weak, the gastrocnemius may likewise appear to be weak when it is not. Thus, the test may be falsely positive. These muscles (primarily the hamstrings) are fixators of the knee during the test and, ideally, should be tested for normal strength prior to testing the gastrocnemius. Pain should not be caused at the contact sites during testing.

Myofascial syndrome

Stretch test: The supine patient fully extends the leg with the foot kept in dorsiflexion (extension). The examiner pushes (without patient resistance) the forefoot into greater dorsal extension (cranially) while pulling the heel downward (caudally). Ideally, a 15°, or more in athletes, increase in extension should be noted. An extension less than 10°, when there is no evidence of mechanical restriction in the ankle mortise, indicates a shortening of the gastrocnemius.

A differential diagnosis is made between shortening of the gastrocnemius and the soleus by flexing the leg at the knee. Knee flexion relaxes the gastrocnemius and allows the stretch to be concentrated more at the soleus.

PIR: The point of departure is from the dorsiflexed (stretched) position as described above. The patient gently contracts the muscle by plantar flexing the foot. In the relaxation phase, the examiner gently pushes the foot back into extension.

Frequently found associated disorders

Hypertonic and chronic muscle shortening conditions are frequently noted. This is very common following ankle trauma. The gastrocnemius has a contractile length of about 3–4 cm. The quadriceps, in comparison, have about a 15 cm contractile length. A minor shortening of 1 cm is very significant for this muscle. During the recovery phase following ankle injury, the patient walks with the foot kept in a neutral position. Flexion and extension components are significantly reduced. Over time, the foot muscles, but most especially the gastrocnemius and soleus shorten. The shortening can lead to firing of the muscle prior to the mid-stance phase during gait and cause over-pronation of the foot. These may also lead to inhibition of the anterior tibialis and, occasionally, the extensor digitorum longus. Flat footedness and calcaneal spurs may also result. This pattern can also be reversed: inhibition of the anterior leg muscles that leads to a reactive contraction of the gastrocnemius.

Compression weakness

Lesion of the S1 root (disc L5/S1) leads to weakness of the gastrocnemius (together with that of the flexor hallucis longus, Mm. peroneus longus and brevis) (Patten 1998, Walther 2000).

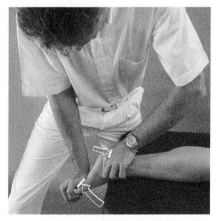

Test of gastrocnemius (Leaf 1996)

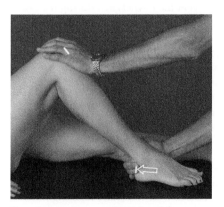

Test of gastrocnemius (both heads)

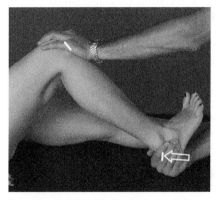

Test of medial head of gastrocnemius

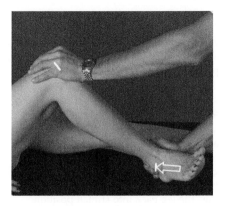

Test of lateral head of gastrocnemius

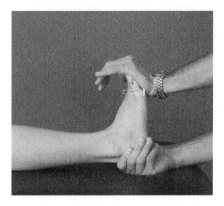

Extension and PIR of gastrocnemius: contraction phase

Anatomy

Origin: At the lateral surface of the ilium posterior to the linea glutea posterior, from the thoracolumbar fascia, the lateral margin of the sacrum and coccyx and the sacrotuberal ligament.

Course: Converging diagonally downwards and laterally towards the femur.

Insertion: On the lower third at the gluteal tuberosity of the femur. The upper two-thirds of the muscle radiate more laterally and insert into the iliotibial tract of the fascia lata. This is significant in that the fascia lata inserts laterally at the tibia and fibula. Thus, both the gluteus maximus and the TFL aid in providing lateral stability to the knee.

Action

With the pelvis fixed, extension and lateral rotation of the femur and with the femur fixed, it will extend (straighten up) the pelvis on the hip. The uppermost fibres can aid in the abduction of the femur. The greatest extension effect is noted with long strides and when climbing stairs. As noted above, it aids in stabilization of the lateral knee. When all muscles are evaluated individually, it should be the strongest single muscle in the body. As a consequence, stabilization of the SI joint is of great clinical significance.

Signs of weakness: Visible atrophy is observed in the 'flaccid butt' syndrome. Difficulties include standing up from a seated position where there is the tendency to 'crawl' up the thigh using the hands. Anterior rotation of the ilium, a high hip and, lateral knee instability (genu varum) on the side of weakness are also common.

Test

Position: The prone patient flexes the knee by more than 90° so that the synergistic hamstrings are taken out of the test. This is followed by the femur being maximally extended at the hip to a point just before the pelvis lifts from the table. Patient capacity may vary significantly.

Stabilization: The pelvis should be stabilized to avoid excess rotation. Usually, excess rotation is caused by to great an elevation from the table surface. Often, when the patient senses weakness, extension of the knee to bring the hamstrings into play is common. In these cases, the knee must be held in a flexed position to prevent their synergism during the test.

Test contact: At the distal thigh just above the popliteal space.

Patient: Extends the thigh (pushes it backwards) as much as possible.

Examiner: Attempts to depress the leg towards the table.

Test errors, precautions: The test position must be maintained. Attempts by the patient to extend the knee must be restricted. When aiding the patient in keeping the knee flexed, it is imperative that counter-resistance to knee extension not be made. By forcefully resisting extension, the quadriceps muscles are brought into the test and, while not hip extensions, facilitate 'locking down' of the coxofemoral joint.

Myofascial syndrome

Stretch test: The supine patient maximally flexes the leg to be tested at the hip and the knee.

The contralateral leg remains extended and resting on the table.

PIR: The patient is asked to fully exhale and hold it. Starting from the point of maximum stretch, the patient is instructed to gradually extend the hip of the flexed leg. This is followed by the patient slowly breathing in while the examiner gently brings the leg back into stretch position.

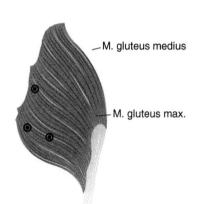

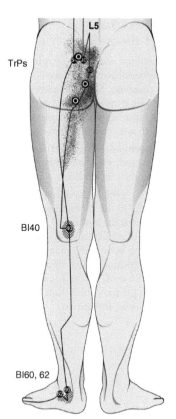

Gluteus maximus including trigger points

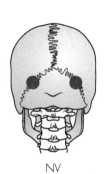

NV

Trigger points and effective distal points

Motor function innervation: Inferior gluteal nerve, L5, S1
Visceroparietal segment, TS line: L3
Rib pump: Intercostal space, costotransverse joint 7, 10
Organ: Gonads
Meridian: Pericardium (Circulation-Sex)
Nutrients: Vitamins A, B3, C, E, PUFA, Se, Zn, Mg
SRS: T5–T12, L1–L5, S1–S3

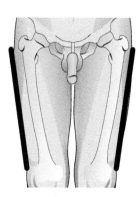

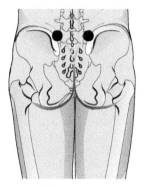

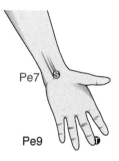

NL anterior   NL posterior

Frequently found associated disorders

A bilateral functional weakness coupled with lumbar hyperlordosis and facet imbrication is common. Micro-fixations of the upper cervical spine causing reflex weakness of the gluteus maximus muscles (Goodheart 1979) are also common.

Functional weakness will predispose SI joint dysfunction and, via the iliotibial tract insertion, lateral knee instability.

Inhibition of the gluteus maximus can lead to hypertonus of the piriformis muscle or a strain-counterstrain lesion and, thus, the development of a piriformis syndrome. Nerve compression symptoms may be confused with pseudoradicular symptoms arising from the SI joint. When, for some reason, there is a primary inhibition of the piriformis muscle, the gluteus maximus, as a consequence, may become hypertonic.

The insidious and somewhat difficult to evaluate spondylogenic reflexes (Sutter 1975) can lead to complex pictures of pain. Using AK differential diagnosis methods, these can be more easily analysed.

Compression weakness: In some rare cases, this can be caused by hypertonus of the piriformis muscle that entraps the inferior gluteal nerve at the infrapiriform foramen. Conversely, weakness of the gluteus maximus may cause reflexive hypertonicity of the piriformis and, eventually, piriformis syndrome. A more complicated, reciprocal dysfunction may be found between the gluteus maximus and the piriformis and they will negatively feed off one-another in a vicious, never ending merry-go-round of imbalance.

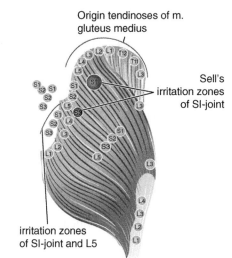

Origin tendinoses of m. gluteus medius

Sell's irritation zones of SI-joint

irritation zones of SI-joint and L5

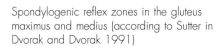

Spondylogenic reflex zones in the gluteus maximus and medius (according to Sutter in Dvorak and Dvorak 1991)

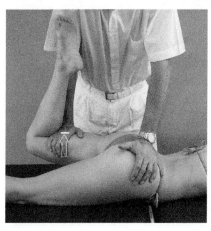

Test of the gluteus maximus

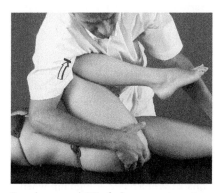

Stretch test and PIR of gluteus maximus in supine position

Anatomy

Origin: From the lateral surface of the ilium (anterior three-quarters of the iliac crest).

Course: In a fan-like pattern on the lateral surface of the ileum. The posterior bundle of fibres cross over and loop under the anterior fibres. The much bigger gluteus maximus overlies the posterior part and the anterior insertion is covered by the tensor fasciae latae. In the deepest layer lies the gluteus minimus. The gluteus minimus is always active during testing of the gluteus medius and distinguishing one from the other in the test is impossible.

Insertion: At the lateral surface of the greater trochanter.

Action

The anterior fibres flex the thigh and rotate it medially, while the posterior fibres extend and rotate laterally.

All fibres abduct the thigh. When the leg is fixed, all fibres pull the pelvis towards the same side of contraction. In a one legged stance it stabilizes the pelvis laterally.

Signs of weakness: A high hip when standing and an excessive medial shift of the pelvis during the stance phase of gait (waddling gait). When standing on the leg on the side of the weak muscle, the pelvis cannot be maintained horizontally (Trendelenburg's sign).

Test

Classic test: (Kendall 1983)

Position: Patient is side-lying with the leg to be tested uppermost. The knee is fully extended and slightly externally rotated, then abducted not more than 45° from the midline. The lower leg is flexed at the knee to aid in trunk stability during the test.

Stabilization: The bent lower leg provides most of the stabilization. The examiner must concentrate on keeping the pelvis in a neutral position. No anterior or posterior rotation of the pelvis should be allowed.

Test contact: On the distal, lateral aspect of the upper leg. The contact position may

vary a bit (from the mid to lower leg) according to the strength of the patient.

Patient: From the start position of about 45° abduction, the patient attempts to further abduct the leg by elevating it away from the table.

Examiner: Resists by depressing the leg toward the table. Due to the long lever it is important that the examiner offers resistance in a vector that follows the natural arc of motion of the leg.

Alternative test position

The supine patient lies with the side to be tested close to the edge of the table. The leg is abducted to about 45° from the midline and slightly externally rotated. At this point it is extended (dropped below the edge of the table) by approximately 20°. External rotation and extension at the hip helps to exclude synergistic activity of the m. tensor fasciae latae.

Stabilization: The examiner takes up a position at the end of the table and stabilization is made on the lateral aspect of the opposite leg.

Test contact: On the distal, lateral aspect of the tested leg.

Patient: Abducts and slightly depress the leg.

Examiner: Resists by trying to adduct and slightly flex the leg at the hip in a direction that will bring the leg just above the surface of the table and towards the midline of the body.

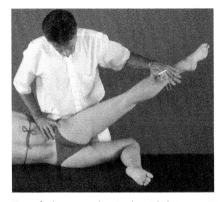

Test of gluteus medius in the side-lying position

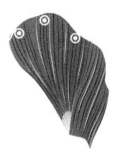

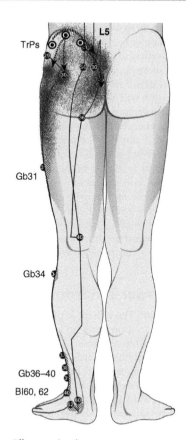

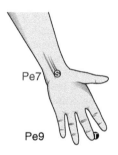

Effective distal points

Motor function innervation: Superior gluteal nerve, L4, L5, S1
Visceroparietal segment, TS line: L5
Rib pump: Intercostal space, costotransverse joint 4, 5, 9, 10
Organ: Gonads, uterus, prostate
Meridian: Pericardium (circulation-sex)
Nutrients: Vitamins A, B3, C, E, PUFA, Mg, Se, Zn
SRS:
Anterior fibres: Thoracic spine
Posterior fibres: L1–L4

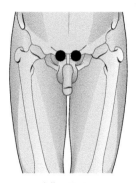

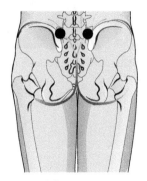

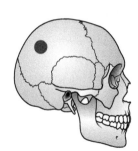

NL anterior   NL posterior   NV

Testing errors, precautions: Poor stabilization of the opposite leg leads to body sideslip during the test. Any medial rotation of the leg or flexion of the hip will bring the tensor fascia lata into the test. Knee flexion will allow contraction of the hamstring muscles and, while not strongly synergistic to the gluteus medius, tend to 'lock down' the hip joint and make accurate testing more difficult.

Functional weakness of the muscle can, under some circumstances (especially in strong individuals), only be observed by testing the patient in the classic, side-lying position. Careful note should be made of the testing differentials mentioned below in the 'compression weakness' section.

Myofascial syndrome

Stretch test: The patient is placed in a side-lying position with the lower leg flexed at the hip and knee. The trunk is rotated slightly backwards for greater stability during the test. The upper leg is maintained extended in the knee and moved forward to flex the hip. The leg should be approximately perpendicular to the body. At this point it is moved downward passing the upper edge of the table until movement is naturally restricted by muscle tension.

PIR: In the side-lying position and with the muscle is fully stretched, the patient is told to gently lift the leg only a few inches. No resistance is offered by the examiner. The relaxation phase follows where the weight of the leg itself is used to elongate the muscle.

Frequently found associated disorders

Compression weakness: Compression of the superior gluteal nerve (L4, L5, S1), leads to gluteus medius dysfunction and may be found in conjunction with the piriformis syndrome. Weakness caused by the piriformis syndrome is often only noted when the test is made in the supine position. Here the piriformis is also contracted in order to stabilize the SI joint and compromises the nerve. Gluteus medius weakness is less evident in the classic, side-lying postion as the piriformis muscle is not contracting to stabilize the SI joint.

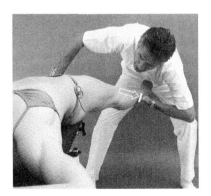

Test of the gluteus medius in the supine position

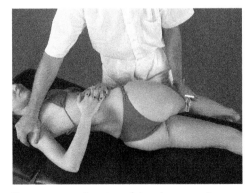

Post-isometric relaxation of the gluteus medius

Anatomy

Origin: In a fan-like pattern from the lateral wing of the ilium in an area found between the inferior and anterior gluteal lines. The posterior fibres originate from the margin of the greater sciatic notch.

Course: Passing under the gluteus medius and ending at the anterior margin of the greater trochanter.

Insertion: Anterior margin of the greater trochanter and the hip joint capsule.

Action

Abduction and medial rotation of the femur and aids in flexion of the hip.

Test

The minimus cannot be effectively differentiated from the gluteus medius.

Myofascial syndrome

Stretch test, PIR: As for the gluteus medius.

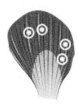

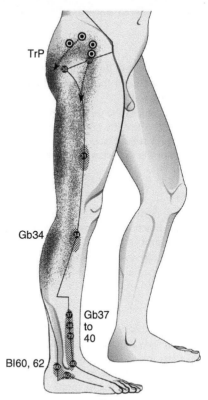

TrP

Gb34

Gb37
to
40

Bl60, 62

Trigger points and effective distal points

Motor function innervation:
Superior gluteal nerve, L4, L5, S1
Visceroparietal segment, TS line: L5
Rib pump: Intercostal space, costotransverse
joint 4, 5, 9, 10
Organ: Gonads (uterus, prostate)
Meridian: Pericardium (circulation-sex)
Nutrients: Vitamins A, B3, C, E, PUFA, Mg,
Se, Zn
SRS: T4–T12

Anatomy

Origin: Just lateral to the symphysis pubis on the anterior side of the inferior aspect of the pubic ramus.

Insertion: Distal to the medial condyle on the proximal part of the medial surface of the tibia. The tendon lies posterior to the tendon of the sartorius at the pes anserinus.

Action

At the hip it adducts and flexes the thigh. At the knee it acts as a flexor and medial (internal) rotator of the leg.

Signs of weakness: A posterior rotation of the ilium, medial knee instability (genu valgus) and pain on palpation of the muscle.

Test

Classic test: action at the knee.

For this test the examiner must follow several steps in order to arrive at the proper test position. The patient is prone with the femur abducted to about 30° and medially rotated about 20°. The foot will rotate away from the midline. The knee is lifted from the table and supported there on the examiner's thigh to keep the hip in extension. When the leg is comfortably elevated and supported, the knee is flexed to approximately 45° and the tibia medially rotated so that the toes point towards the midline.

Stabilization: The leg must be kept in extension at the hip during the test. This is achieved by placing the patient's thigh on the examiner's, whose flexed knee rests on the examing table. The stabilizing hand holds the patient's thigh in place. Great downward pressure is exerted by the patient as the rectus femoris and psoas muscles contract during the resistance phase.

Test contact: On the distal, medial aspect of the patient's lower leg close to the posterior aspect of the medial malleolus.

Patient: Flexes the lower leg.

Examiner: Resists by attempting to extend the leg following the natural arc of the leg about the knee. Any attempt to externally rotate the femur should be avoided.

Test of the action at the hip (Beardall 1981)

In certain texts, the gracilis muscle was described as 'adductor gracilis'. The Beardall test evaluates this adductor capacity.

Position: The leg of the supine patient is kept in a neutral position and in line with the body so that there is no abduction or adduction. The femur is rotated internally.

Stabilization: Internal, distal aspect of the opposite leg.

Test contact: Internal and slightly anterior, distal aspect of the tested leg.

Patient: Adducts the tested leg by drawing it towards the stabilized leg.

Examiner: Attempts to abduct the leg by pulling the legs apart.

Test errors, precautions: In the supine position – poor stabilization of the contralateral leg.

In the prone test, pain may be caused by undue stress on the structures surrounding the knee. This is primarily due to a less than optimum stabilization or excessive contact pressure and failing to keep the leg elevated above the table surface.

Myofascial syndrome

Stretch test: The supine patient is positioned so that the leg to be examined is close to the edge of the table. The leg is then abducted, laterally rotated and slightly extended at the hip. The non-tested leg must be fixed on the table in a neutral position.

PIR: Starting from the stretched position the patient is asked to take a deep breath and hold it, while slowly adducting the leg. In the relaxation phase, the patient breathes out while the examiner elongates the muscle into the stretch position.

Frequently found associated disorders

Hypoadrenia of the adrenal glands is a common cause of gracilis weakness that may cause an SI joint lesion due to a posterior rotation of the ilium. Instability and pain at the medial knee are also sequelae.

Compression weakness: Obturator syndrome caused by pregnancy and trauma compromising the obturator canal.

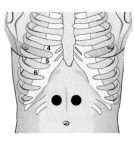

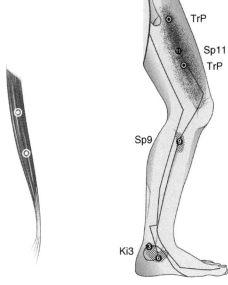

Motor function innervation:
Obturator nerve, L2, L3, L4
Visceroparietal segment, TS line:
T9
SRS: L4
Rib pump: Intercostal space, costotransverse joints 6, 8
Meridian: Pericardium (circulation Sex)
Organ: Adrenal glands
Nutrients: Vitamins B3, B5, B6, B12, folic acid, adrenal extract, ginseng

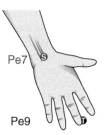

Trigger points, effective distal points

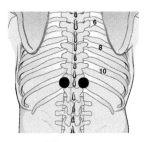

NL anterior

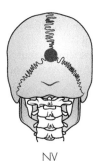

NL posterior

NV

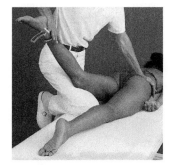

Gracilis test according to Kendall, Goodheart and Walther

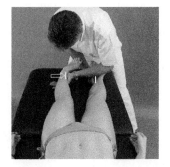

Gracilis test according to Beardall

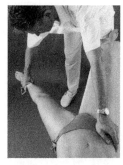

PIR of the gracilis stretch phase

Hamstrings (ischiocrural muscles)

Anatomy

Origin: Semitendinosus and semimembranosus: By a common tendon together with the biceps femoris at the ischial tuberosity.

Biceps femoris (long head): Ischial tuberosity and sacrotuberous ligament.

Biceps femoris (short head): Lateral lip of the linea aspera of the femur.

Insertion: Semimembranous: At the medial tibial condyle but also with three fibrous expansions. One tract of fibres strengthens the knee joint capsule from behind by coursing vertically and laterally. A second tract of fibres runs over and covers the popliteus muscle to end at the linea m. solei and a third unites with the fibres of the medial collateral ligament and fascia.

Semitendinosus: Having the most posterior tendon, it forms the pes anserinus together with the tendons of the semimembranosus, sartorius and gracilis. All the tendons of the pes anserinus have a common insertion at the medial surface of the tibia.

Biceps femoris muscle: Lateral tibial condyle and lateral part of the head of the fibula.

Action

Flexion of the knee joint and extension of the hips and they help in maintaining an upright position when walking.

A secondary function of the hamstrings is rotation of the hip and knee joints with internal rotation being made primarily by the medial hamstrings and external rotation by the lateral hamstrings.

Signs of weakness: Imbalance between the medial and lateral hamstrings may lead to a rotational dysfunction causing medial or lateral knee instability and, ultimately, genu valgum or varum. Anterior ilium rotation and a slight elevation of the pelvis on the involved side may also be noted.

Test

Position: The knee is flexed no more than 60° and with very strong patients no more than 45°.

For a general test of both medial and lateral divisions, no rotation is imparted on the femur or lower leg.

The medial hamstrings are tested with a 30° internal rotation of the thigh and for the lateral hamstrings, 30° of external rotation.

Stabilization: Somewhere in the area of the pelvis, trying not to contact the SI joint in order to avoid a rare, examiner induced, accidental TL. Stabilization is not critical as the prone body position is more than adequate for patient stability.

Alternative stabilization contacts may be made. The hand may be placed slightly above the iliac crest, or, when there is a tendency for cramping, the fist may compress the hamstring belly. Both involve a limited risk of undesirable TL. As well, one should be aware that the pressure on the muscle belly by the fisted hand might cause a type of challenge provocation.

Test contact: With a broad contact on the calcaneus and the Achilles tendon, taking care not to provoke pain. A more proximal contact over the soleus and gastrocnemius muscles may be used in weaker patients.

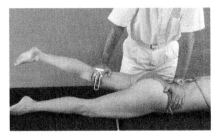

Hamstring test – function of the proximal fibres

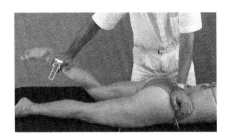

Group hamstring test

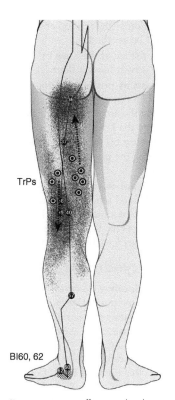

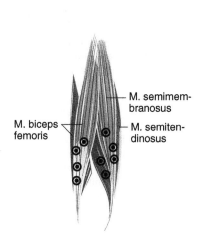

M. biceps femoris

M. semimem-branosus

M. semiten-dinosus

TrPs

BI60, 62

Trigger points, effective distal points

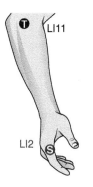

T

LI11

LI2

S

Motor function innervation: Sciatic nerve, L4, L5, S1, S2
Visceroparietal segment, TS line: L1
Rib pump: Intercostal space, 10th costotransverse joint
SRS: T12, L1 for biceps femoris, L5 for semimembranosus, S2 for semitendinosus
Meridian: Large intestine
Organ: Rectum
Nutrients: Vitamin E, calcium, magnesium, l-glutamine

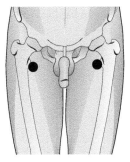

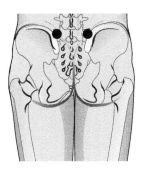

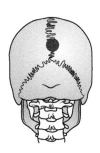

NL anterior   NL posterior   NV

Unwanted irritation of the tendon and its insertion should be avoided.

Patient: Flexes the leg at the knee by pressing firmly upwards with the heel.

Examiner: Resists by pushing the foot inferiorly and then down towards the table surface following the arc of motion of the leg when bending the knee.

The extensor effect on the hips can be assessed by testing the proximal fibres as illustrated above.

Test errors, precautions: A synergistic recruitment is allowed when the precise testing vector is not maintained and by the patient lifting the pelvis. Knee flexion greater than 60° may lead to cramping.

Myofascial syndrome

Stretch test (evaluating adverse tension): The supine patient extends the leg and lifts it from the table surface, as in the straight leg raise test (Lasègue). A shortening of the hamstrings may be concluded if the hip can only flex to 80° or less. Included in this figure is the 10° of posterior rotation afforded by the pelvis. Any pain felt at the buttocks and along the back of the leg during stretching cannot be immediately differentiated from root irritation originating in the lumbar spine. Pain from root irritation is usually more pronounced distally, but even this is not always the case. When trigger points are present in the gastrocnemius, additional dorsal flexion of the foot may be used in cases of shortening and will increase the feeling of tension and pain in the back of the knee and calf.

There are several ways in which to differentiate between hamstring shortening and a nerve root involvement. One of the best is to begin evaluating for trigger points and post-isometric relaxation

problems in the myofascia of the hamstrings. When found and treated, a significant change in hip flexion ability will be noted. When nerve root irritation is present, treatment of the trigger points and PIR therapy will produce no improvement in flexion capacity.

PIR: From the stretch position, the patient is instructed to take and hold an inspiration while gradually bringing the leg down to the table surface. The relaxation phase follows with the patient breathing out as the examiner slowly brings the leg back to the stretch position and slightly beyond. Breathing out tends to contract the abdominal muscles and straighten the lumbar spine by retroflexing the pelvis. Since the abdominals are synergistic to the hamstrings, breathing in tends to inhibit both the hamstrings and the abdominals, leading to a greater anterior tilting of the pelvis.

Frequently found associated disorders

Functional hamstring weakness is often found as a consequence of SI lesions. In all cases of knee instability, the hamstrings should always be considered as a contributing factor. Bilateral hamstring weakness may be indicative of sacral or sacrococcygeal restrictions related to the craniosacral mechanism. These are defined in AK as sacral and sacrococcegeal inspiration or expiration assist faults.

As well, lower bowel dysfunction and/ or haemorrhoids may cause bilateral weakness or hyper-reactive reactions of the hamstring muscles.

Compression weakness: S1 root syndrome (intervertebral foramen L5/S1), piriformis syndrome, iliolumbar ligament syndrome.

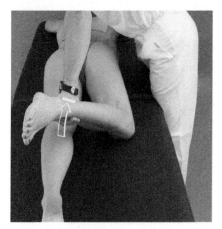

Lateral hamstring test

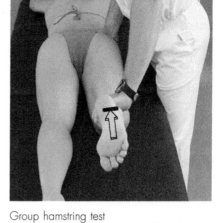

Group hamstring test

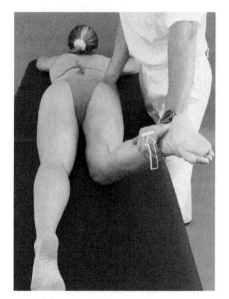

Medial hamstring test

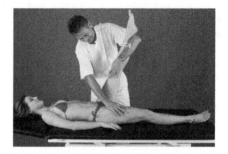

PIR: contraction with expiration

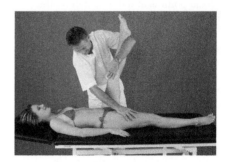

PIR: extension with inspiration

Anatomy

Origin: Superior two-thirds of the iliac fossa from an area close to the SI joint, lumbosacral and iliolumbar ligaments.

Course: Converges and passes over the superior ramus of the pubic bone and under the inguinal ligament. Here the muscle usually fuses with the psoas to form a common, flattened tendon.

Insertion: Together with the psoas at the lesser trocanter.

Action

The muscle mainly flexes, adducts and slight medially rotates the femur (Palastanga and Field 1989, Schiebler and Schmidt 1999). Some sources (Walther 2000, Travell and Simons 1992) report a slight lateral rotation of the femur is possible. Since the muscle inserts medially to the central pivot point of the hip joint, internal rotation is a more likely than external. By altering the relationship of the hip pivot, as in flexion, the insertion angle of the muscle changes. Thus, with the thigh flexed and abducted, contraction of the muscle will cause flexion, lateral rotation and adduction. Standing, where the fixed point is at the insertion on the femur, contraction will rotate the pelvis anteriorly.

Signs of weakness: The ilium will tend to rotate posterior causing a functional short leg, a shortened forward step and a pronounced 'kick' or 'flick' of the lower leg when walking. An external rotation or 'flaring' of the pelvis on the opposite side of weakness may also be noted. The flaring is predominantly due to compensatory activity on the side of weakness. The oblique abdominal muscles will increase their activity and cause the pelvis to rotate internally. The pelvis on the opposite side will compensate by flaring externally.

Test

Position: The leg of the supine patient is laterally rotated, extended at the knee, and placed in 45°, or more, of abduction. This is followed by flexing the leg at the hip about 60–70°. A more pronounced flexion of the leg differentiates this test from that of the psoas muscle.

Stabilization: The pelvis on the opposite side.

Test contact: Medially, on the proximal part of lower leg, just below the knee. The exact position may vary according to patient strength.

Patient: First, the patient must be able to hold the leg in the test position. This is followed by elevating the leg in a diagonal direction by flexing and slightly adducting the leg at the hip.

Examiner: Attempts to depress the leg toward the table. The resistance vector should be downward and slightly lateral towards the table. This will follow the natural arc of movement of the leg made by iliacus muscle contraction.

Test errors, precautions: Differentiation from the psoas muscle is made solely by noting a greater flexion and abduction of the hip joint. Accuracy in differentiation will ultimately depend upon examiner precision. The tested leg must be brought into the specific start position and supported there by the examiner. This eliminates pre-testing fatigue of the muscle due to the weight of the leg. In some cases it is best that a 'rehearsal' of the patient's resisting movement is made prior to performing the actual test procedure.

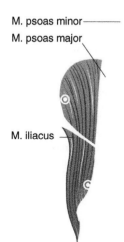

M. psoas minor————

M. psoas major

M. iliacus ——

Motor function innervation: L2, L3, L4
Visceroparietal segment, TS line: T11, T12
Rib pump: Intercostal space, costotransverse joint 4, 7, 12
SRS: L1–L5, SIJ
Organ: Kidneys
Nutrients: Vitamins A and E
Meridian: Kidneys

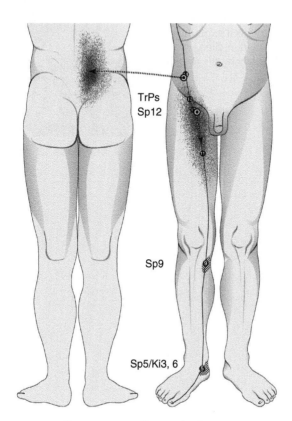

TrPs
Sp12

Sp9

Sp5/Ki3, 6

Trigger points, effective distal points

Myofascial syndrome

Stretch test: Since the psoas and iliacus cannot be adequately separated from each other, the stretch test will encompass both muscles. The supine patient lies with the leg to be tested hanging over the end of the table. The opposite leg is flexed at the hip and the examiner stabilizes the patient's pelvis and lumbar spine by holding the knee. The tested leg naturally flexes at the knee and is allowed to hang down extending the hip entirely by its own weight. Should any overstretching of the muscle be made, trigger point pain can be provoked.

PIR: From the stretched position, the patient holds an inspiration for about 10 s and slowly lifts the opposite leg, while keeping the lower leg naturally flexed at the knee. Any extension of the knee will stimulate activity of the synergistic rectus femoris muscle and may reduce the therapeutic effect. During the relaxation phase, the patient slowly breathes out while the flexed leg is allowed to gradually drop back to the start position. Elongation of the muscle is made solely by the weight of the extended leg.

Frequently found associated disorders

On the side of muscle shortening the ilium will tend to rotate anteriorly. On the weak side, the ilium will tend to rotate posteriorly. Classic 'clicking hip' and pseudo-ovarian pains may also be noted.

Cause for compression: Trigger points, as well as, increased tension and hypertrophy within the muscle may lead to nerve entrapment between the inguinal ligament and the iliopsoas/iliacus muscle bundle. Entrapment of the lateral femoral cutaneous nerve of the anterior thigh may ensue with corresponding paraesthesia (Lewit 1992, Travell and Simons 1992).

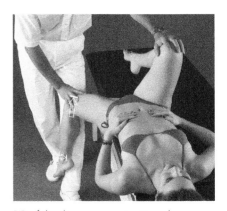

PIR of the iliopsoas, contraction phase

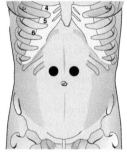

NL anterior

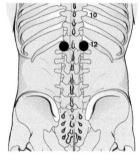

NL posterior

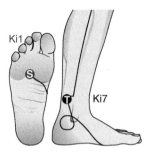

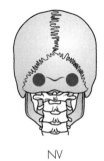

NV

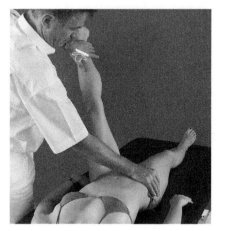

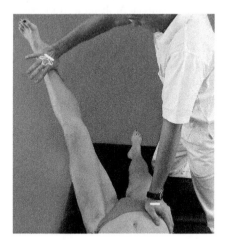

Iliacus test. The test position on the right is more ergonomic

Anatomy

Origin: Medial two thirds of the infraspinous fossa.

Course: Converges medial to lateral.

Insertion: Middle facet of the greater tubercle of humerus with some fibres into the shoulder joint capsule.

Action

Lateral (external) rotation of the humerus. Together with the teres minor it is one of the few dorsally oriented stabilizers of the head of the humerus. The stabilizing effect is predominant when the arm is abducted alongside the trunk. Interestingly, the upper fibres aid more in abducting and the lower fibres more in adducting the arm.

Signs of weakness: When standing, the relaxed, hanging arm may have an increased medial rotation, seen both at the hand and elbow. Atrophy of the muscle is easily noted by a lack of substance that can be palpated in the area just inferior to the spine of the scapula. A 'dishing' of the soft tissue is easily seen.

Test

Position: With the elbow flexed to 90°, the humerus is laterally rotated to its natural limit and abducted to approximately 90°.

Stabilization: On the medial elbow, taking care to avoid finger contact on the acupuncture drainage point TH10.

Test contact: Close to the wrist or on the dorsum of the distal forearm.

Patient: Laterally (externally) rotates the humerus by pushing the wrist backwards.

Examiner: Resistance is made to internally rotate the humerus following the arc of motion as the forearm moves about a fixed point at the elbow.

By reducing the abduction of the arm to a point between 45°, and less than 90°, the more superior fibres of the muscle are tested. Conversely, testing made with 90° of abduction should isolate the more inferior fibres.

Test errors, precautions: A less than maximal lateral rotation of the humerus along with a poor medial stabilization at the elbow are the two more frequently noted errors. Pain elicited by a too enthusiastic grip of either the testing or stabilizing hand may also falsify findings. During the testing procedure, observe for compensatory movements made at the shoulder joint. Compensatory movements are dynamic signs of recruitment due to possible muscle weakness.

If the patient tends to deviate too far from the test position, it may be necessary to change the position by placing the stabilizing hand on the patient's shoulder. Thus, the patient's elbow will rest on the more stabile and stronger forearm of the examiner.

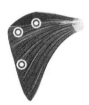

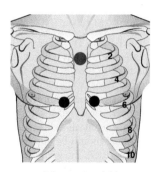

NL anterior; NV

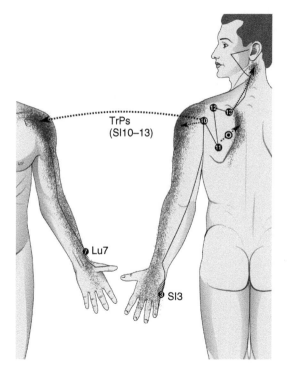

TrPs
(SI10–13)

Lu7

SI3

Trigger points, effective distal points

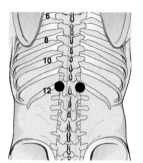

NL posterior

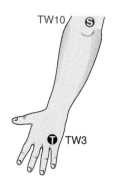

TW10

TW3

Motor function innervation: Suprascapular nerve, C(4), C5, C6
Rib pump: Intercostal space, costotransverse joint 1, 2, 10
Organ: Thymus
Nutrients: Se, Zn, Cu, antioxidants, thymus extracts
Meridian: TW

Myofascial syndrome

Stretch test: The humerus is medially rotated as far as it will naturally go and the hand is moved behind and placed close to the opposite shoulder blade in order to stretch the superior fibres. The more caudal fibres are stretched when the arm is pulled across the anterior chest wall. Both positions should be applied and the one that produces the greatest radiating pain is selected for therapy.

PIR: Starting from the most painful of the above stretch positions, the patient slowly draws the arm back to the neutral position at the trunk. During the relaxation phase, the examiner returns the limb to the initial stretch position and, then, slightly beyond to increase the stretch a bit more.

Frequently found associated disorders

Weakness leads to reflex hypertonicity and shortening of the subscapularis muscle. Extremely painful trigger points will also be noted in the subscapularis resulting in a reduced ability to abduct and flex the humerus and can be an early warning sign for adhesive capsulitis or 'frozen shoulder'. In the more advanced stages, when becoming 'frozen', the scapula will begin lateral movement during the very early stages of arm abduction.

Compression weakness: Cervical root syndrome due to irritation of the 5th cervical nerve as it passes through the intervertebral foramen at C4/C5 and from entrapment of the suprascapular nerve as it traverses through the scapular notch. Aberrant movement patterns and instability of the scapula are the primary causes of suprascapular nerve entrapment.

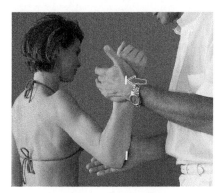

Infraspinatus test: superior fibres

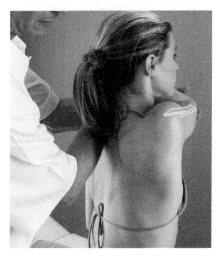

PIR of the inferior infraspinatus fibres:
contraction phase

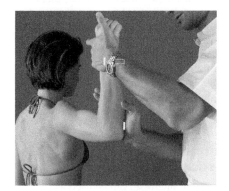

Infraspinatus test: inferior fibres

Anatomy

They are unlike most muscles in that they have no attachment to bone, but to the tendons of the flexor digitorum profundus proximally and, distally, to the extensor tendons.

Origin: Interosseus dorsalis I: Radial head and proximal half of the ulnar margin of the 1st metacarpal bone.

Interosseus dorsalis I: Ulnar head and radial side of the 2nd metacarpal bone.

Interossei dorsales II, II, IV: From the opposed surfaces of the 2nd to 5th metacarpal bones.

Insertion: The tendons radiate into the dorsal aponeurosis of the fingers and insert at the base of the proximal phalanx.

I: Radial side of the index finger.
II: Radial side of the middle finger.
III: Ulnar side of the middle finger.
IV: Ulnar side of the ring finger.

Action

I: Radial abduction of the index finger.
II: Radial abduction of the middle finger.
III: Ulnar abduction of the middle finger.
IV: Ulnar abduction of the ring finger.

Signs of weakness: Inability or difficulty in spreading the fingers.

Test

The spreading or splaying capacity of the 2nd to 4th fingers is tested, as well as radial and ulnar abduction of the middle finger. First the index finger and then the ring finger are stabilized. The test can normally only be fully interpreted by comparing the results with those of the patient's other, healthy hand.

Myofascial syndrome

Stretch test: The fingers are individually spread apart from each other in order to stretch the separate divisions of the muscle.

Causes for compression: The digital cutaneous branches of the ulnar and median nerves can be irritated by trigger points and hypertonicity of the interossei, leading to hypoaesthesia and dysaesthesia of the relevant fingers. Proximal and distal compression of the ulnar nerve may be derived from the sulcus ulnaris or ulnar tunnel syndromes and trigger points in the opponens digiti minimi. All more proximal entrapments, ranging from the neck to the axilla of the arm, including the tunnels around the elbow, will cause concomitant weakness of these muscles. Differential diagnosis is made by TL along the route of the nerves in order to locate the primary entrapment.

Frequently found associated disorders

The dorsal interossei can be used as indicator muscles for C8-root irritation caused by C7/T1 disc protrusion or prolapse.

The importance of the muscles must not be underestimated. These, along with the other intrinsic muscles of the hand, have a very high number of spindle cells that send proprioceptive afferents into the central nervous system. So powerful are they that in spastic patients a simple stroking massage made in the metacarpal spaces will often lead to a relaxation of the whole extremity.

Mm. interossei
dorsales

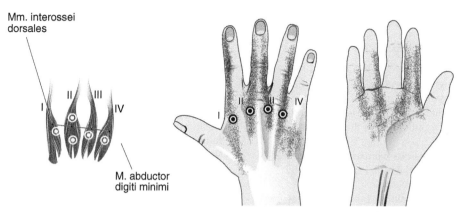

M. abductor
digiti minimi

Trigger points and referred pain from the
dorsal and palmar interossei

Motor function innervation:
Ulnar nerve (C8, T1)

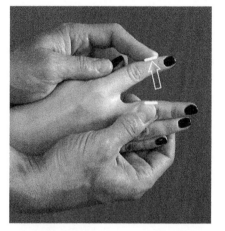

Interosseus dorsalis I

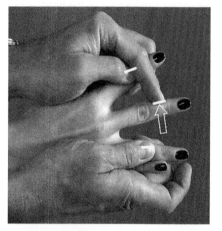

Interosseus dorsalis II

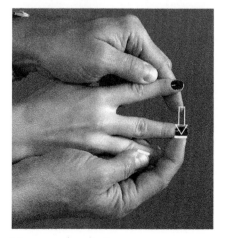

Interosseus dorsalis III

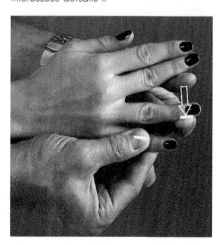

Interosseus dorsalis IV

Mm. interossei palmares

Anatomy

Origin: Interosseus palmaris I: The entire length of the ulnar side of the 2nd metacarpal bone.

Interosseus palmaris II: The entire length of the radial side of the 4th metacarpal bone.

Interosseus palmaris III: The entire length of the radial side of the 5th metacarpal bone.

The muscles lie between the metacarpal bones in the deepest layer of the hand.

Insertion: The tendons insert at the base of the proximal phalanx of 2nd, 4th and 5th fingers and also radiate deeper to insert in the dorsal aponeurosis of the hand.

I: Ulnar side of the index finger.
II: Radial side of the ring finger.
III: Radial side of the little finger.

Action

Adduction of the thumb and index finger toward the middle finger as well as adduction of the ring (4th) finger and little finger toward the middle finger.

Test

Isolating the interosseus palmaris I (ulnar side) is not possible due to very strong synergist activity of the adductor pollicis. However, the other four fingers can be tested. Apposition of the index, ring and little fingers to the middle finger may be made. The fingers not involved in the test remain fixed together by the patient.

Frequently found associated disorders

The muscles can be used as indicator muscles for the motor function root C8 from C8/T1 intervertebral disc lesions.

Mm. interossei
palmares

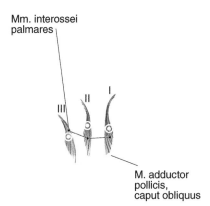

M. adductor
pollicis,
caput obliquus

Motor function innervation: Ulnar nerve (C8, T1)

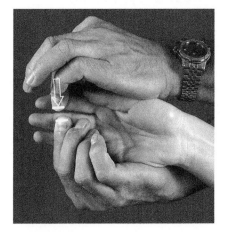

Interosseus palmaris I

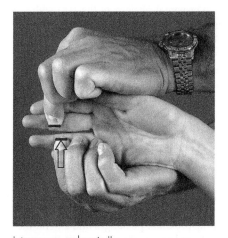

Interosseus palmaris II

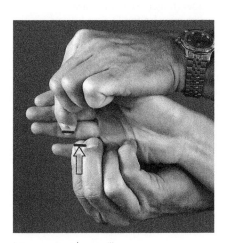

Interosseus palmaris III

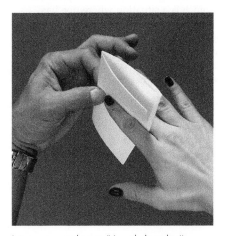

Interosseus palmaris IV and dorsalis II

Mm. lumbricales

Anatomy

Origin: Lumbricales I and II: At the radial side of the tendons of the flexor digitorum profundus of the index and middle fingers.

Lumbricales II und IV: On the facing sides of the tendons of the flexor digitorum profundus of the middle and ring fingers and the ring and little fingers.

Course: From the proximal origin to the distal insertion, lying in the middle compartment of the palmer muscles.

Insertion: Like the interossei, they insert dorsally on the fingers, albeit a bit more distally. Their tendons also radiate into the dorsal aponeurosis at the level of the shaft of the proximal phalanx of the 1st to 5th fingers.

Action

Extension of the middle and terminal phalanx and flexion of the proximal phalanx of the 2nd to 5th fingers.

Signs of weakness: When pathologically weak, a combined deformity occurs causing a hyperextension of the proximal phalanges of the 2nd to 5th fingers together with a hyperflexion of the middle and terminal phalanges. A type of 'claw-hand' deformity will be noted. Normally, weakness causes an inability to flex the proximal phalanges and extend the middle and terminal phalanges at the same time, resulting in a 'tip-pinch' dysfunction. Tip-pinch is a situation where one has difficulty in opposing the tips of the index finger and thumb when trying to pick up and hold small objects. Classically, an individual will have difficulty or be totally unable to hold a newspaper in one hand.

Test

Position: Leaving the thumb out of the test, the fingers are flexed at the metacarpophalangeal joints, keeping the interphalangeal joints in extension. Extension of the hand at the wrist will facilitate the intrinsic muscles making it easier for the examiner to distinguish between strength and weakness.

Stabilization: Fixation of the hand and fingers. The fingers must be maintained in extension and the hand in extension at the wrist.

Test contact: On the palmar and distal surfaces of each proximal phalanx.

Patient: Bends the extended finger at the proximal phalanx as far as possible.

Test errors, precautions: Bending the fingers at the distal phalanxes recruits the short and long finger flexors.

Myofascial syndrome

Stretch test: The proximal phalanges of the 2nd to 5th fingers are extended beyond their normal range while the middle and terminal phalanges are maximally flexed.

PIR: From the stretch position the patient slowly flexes the proximal phalanges while the middle and terminal phalanges are extended. In the relaxation phase the examiner returns the fingers to the stretch position and slightly beyond to further elongate the muscles.

Frequently found associated disorders

Compression weaknesses: The interossei (finger abduction) are indicator muscles for T1 root lesions (Patten 1998).

Lumbricales I and II: Carpal tunnel syndrome and all other proximal compression sites for the median nerve from the scalene, costoclavicular, coracopectoral and pronator teres areas.

Lumbricales III and IV: Compression of the thoracic inlet, sulcus ulnaris syndrome and pisiform hamate syndrome.

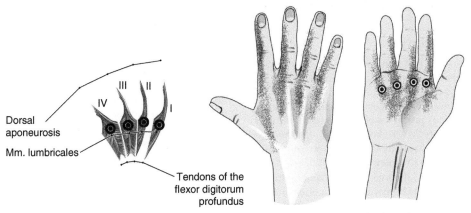

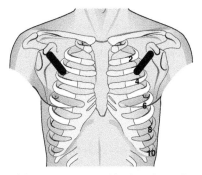

Dorsal
aponeurosis

Mm. lumbricales

Tendons of the
flexor digitorum
profundus

III   II

IV

I

Trigger points, pain transfer from the
lumbricals

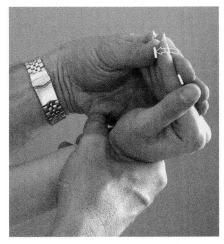

Motor function innervation:
Lumbricals I and II: Median nerve, C(6, 7),
C8, T1
Lumbricals III and IV: Ulnar nerve, C(7), C8,
T1

NL of the interosseus and lumbrical muscles

Lumbricales test

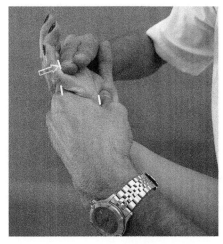

Stretch and PIR of the lumbricals

Anatomy

Origin: From an area broader than any other single muscle, it originates at the iliac crest, the sacrum and from a wide aponeurosis, that encompasses all the spinous processes of the lumbar and lower six thoracic vertebrae. Further origins are derived from the lower three to four ribs and from the inferior angle of the scapula.

Course: Converges superiorly and laterally towards the humerus. The superior most fibres run practically horizontally and the inferior fibres ascend steeply.

Insertion: Proximally, on the medial and anterior humerus at the intertubercular sulcus. The tendon blends with those of the teres major and pectoralis major.

Action

Depression and retraction of the shoulder. Extension, adduction and medial rotation of the humerus. With the arms above the head and the weight of the body suspended by them, this powerful muscle stops the scapula from being pulled away from the trunk. Placing the arms above the head causes a bilateral contraction of the muscles that augments extension of the thoracic spine and increases lumbar lordosis.

Signs of weakness: When standing an elevated and slightly protracted shoulder may be noted on the side of weakness. The palm of the hand may appear to be slightly more laterally rotated, but this is rarely noted.

Test

Position: The elbow is kept fully extended and the humerus put into full medial rotation. The shoulder must not be protracted, otherwise synergistic internal rotators will enter into the test. The starting position should be with the patient's hand slightly behind the greater trochanter as an anterior placement will tend to induce unwanted shoulder flexion. The arm is then abducted 10° (or about a hand's width) from the body.

Stabilization: The free hand is placed on the shoulder to prevent it from lifting and the trunk from leaning to the side being tested.

Test contact: On the dorsal and lateral aspect of the distal forearm, close to the wrist.

Patient: Keeping the elbow in extension, the patient draws the hand towards a point slightly behind the axial midline of the body. Any deviation from this direction may indicate weakness and the test should be repeated until the patient pulls correctly.

Examiner: Resists to primarily abduct and slightly flex the arm. With a resistance vector too posterior, the anterior synergists will automatically enter into the test, eliminating a positive finding.

Test errors, precautions: Any bending of the elbow will recruit the biceps. The best arm position will be slightly behind the trouser seam. No shoulder flexion should be allowed. Pain around the biceps insertion at the elbow during the test is usually a good indication of latissimus weakness.

Myofascial syndrome

Stretch test: The patient sits on a chair with a strong back and is asked to put the arm behind the head so that the hand touches the ear and the cheek on the opposite side. Head flexion in order to achieve this position is not allowed.

PIR: Starting from stretch, a deep inspiration is taken and held for 10 secs while the elbow is moved away from the head against gentle resistance. Relaxation follows where the arm is brought back to the start position while the patient slowly breathes out.

Frequently found associated disorders

Pancreatic dysfunction and thoracic micro-fixations.

Compression weakness: Anterior scalene syndrome.

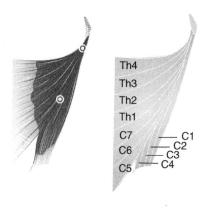

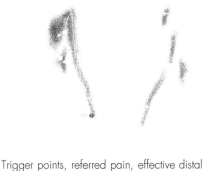

Th4
Th3
Th2
Th1
C7 — C1
C6 — C2
C5 — C3
— C4

Trigger points, referred pain, effective distal points

Spondylogenic reflex zones

Motor function innervation: Thoracodorsal nerve, C6, C7, C8
Visceroparietal segment, TS line: T6
Rib pump: Intercostal space, costotransverse joint 3, 6, 8
Organ: Pancreas
Meridian: Spleen (pancreas)
Nutrients: Vitamins A, B3, Zn, Se, Cr, Mg, PUFA, pancreatic enzymes

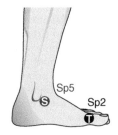

Sp5
Sp2

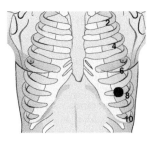

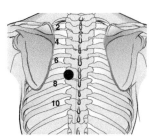

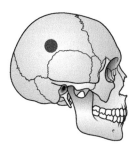

NL anterior

NL posterior

NV

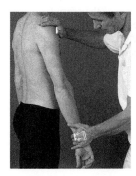
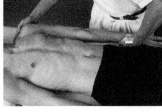
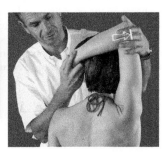

Latissimus dorsi test

Stretch and PIR (contraction phase)

Anatomy

Origin: Transverse processes of atlas and axis and the posterior tubercles of the transverse processes of C3 and C4.

Course: Fibres from the individual origins entwine in a rope-like fashion and converge in an inferior direction. Lying in the second muscle layer of the neck it passes under the trapezius, where it can be palpated. The accessory nerve passes over the top of the muscle.

Insertion: On the superior, medial margin of the scapula between the spine and the superior angle of the scapula.

Action

Elevates the medial, superior angle of the scapula and supports lateral rotation so that the inferior angle moves medially and the glenoid cavity slopes down. The muscle is an antagonist of the upper trapezius with regard to scapular rotation, yet assists it in elevating the scapula and shoulder.

With the scapula fixed, contraction rotates and laterally flexes the cervical spine to the same side. When both sides contract simultaneously, extension of the cervical spine is noted and when the cervical spine is fixed, it aids in shoulder elevation.

Signs of weakness: Observed in the standing position, the superior angle of the scapula may appear to droop and the normal space between the inferior angle and the spine is enlarged compared to the other side. A sudden shift of the scapula, called 'swerve' when lowering the abducted arm is caused by a disharmonious coordination between the rhomboid muscles and the levator scapula. The levator fails to stabilize the scapula during humeral descent and a smooth transition of the arm cannot occur under the combined pulling action of the rhomboids and other shoulder fixators.

Test

Position: Very difficult to differentiate from the rhomboid muscles, the precise testing position is extremely critical. As well, the levator and rhomboids must be isolated from the synergistic action of the upper trapezius. The humerus is placed close in to the trunk, laterally rotated and extended. The elbow should pass well beyond the dorsum of the back. With the elbow maintained in this start position, the patient is instructed to lift the shoulder; automatically restricting any further elevation of the superior, lateral angle of the scapula. This position better isolates the action of the levator on the superior, medial angle of the scapula and aids in reducing any synergistic effects by the upper trapezius. Approximation of the medial scapular border to the spine keeps the rhomboids contracted.

Test contact: One hand covers the area of the upper trapezius muscle, close to the superior, medial angle of the scapula. The palm of the other hand cups the olecranon process and the fingers curl around to grasp the medial elbow.

Patient: In a combined movement, keeps the shoulder elevated and extended while simultaneously drawing the elbow medially and slightly back.

Examiner: Also in a combined movement, pushes down on the shoulder (as medially as is possible) while simultaneously pulling the elbow out to abduct and flex the humerus. The resistance vector should be directed as much as possible at the superior, medial angle of the scapula. Weakness is concluded when the humerus moves laterally and the superior angle of the scapula descends and moves laterally.

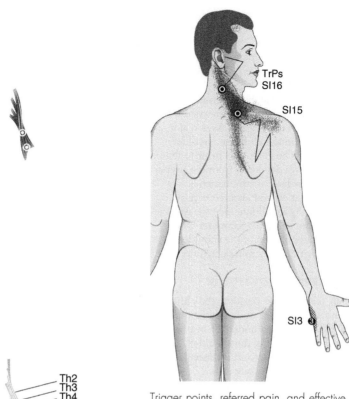

TrPs
SI16
SI15
SI3

Trigger points, referred pain, and effective distal point

Th2
Th3
Th4
Th5

Spondylogenic reflex zones

Motor function innervation: Dorsoscapular nerve, C3, C4, C5
Rib pump: Intercostal space, costotransverse joint 2, 6, 7, 10
Organ: Parathyroid gland
Nutrients: Ca, Mg, vitamin D and other factors of the calcium metabolism
Meridian: Lungs

Test errors, precautions: The rhomboid muscles should be tested for strength prior to the levator scapulae. The rhomboids act as stabilizers of the scapula during the test and if they are weak, the levator scapulae cannot be tested.

General shoulder stabilizers must also be intact. These will include the pectoralis major, middle trapezius and teres major and minor, although all major shoulder muscles should be evaluated prior to the levator test. Any deviation from the proper test position or lack of simultaneous shoulder elevation and arm fixation by the patient may invalidate the test. An imprecise contact by the examiner when attempting depression of the shoulder may allow upper trapezius muscle activity.

Myofascial syndrome

Stretch test: Supine position: the patient's arm and shoulder are pulled down and the hand is fixed in place under the buttocks. The examiner, keeping the shoulder stabilized, lifts, rotates and inclines the head towards the opposite side.

PIR: Starting from the above stretch position, the patient de-rotates the head, while simultaneously extending and laterally flexing it to the opposite side. These movements are made against little resistance. The relaxation phase follows as the examiner returns the head and neck to the stretch position and a bit beyond.

Self-treatment may be performed while sitting on a chair with a good back. The hand on the treatment side grasps the underside of leg of the chair so that the shoulder is held down. The head and neck are forward flexed, then rotated and inclined towards the opposite side.

Alternatively, with the patient in the supine position the arm can be elevated to its maximum height. This causes rotation and depression of the superior, medial angle of the scapula. The arm and scapula are kept fixed in this position. Supporting the head, the examiner moves it into flexion and rotation to the opposite side. The levator scapula should now be under stretch (Dvorák 1991).

Frequently found associated disorders

In a significant number of cases the muscle is riddled with trigger points and is responsible, in large part, for the development of 'cervical spine syndrome'. The formation of trigger points in the muscle may be due to host of problems ranging from psychosomatic factors primarily from emotional stress to overexertion such as carrying heavy loads or from an awkward posture when driving. Infections and other metabolic disturbances also favour the development of trigger points in the muscle. Chronic weakness of the latissimus dorsi (the primary shoulder depressor), can lead to functional shortening of the levator scapula and the formation of trigger points.

Compression weakness: Scapulocostal syndrome and thoracic outlet syndrome (Leaf 1996).

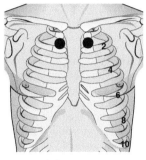

NL anterior

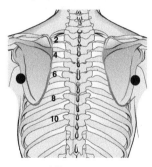

NL posterior

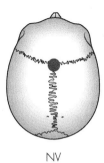

NV

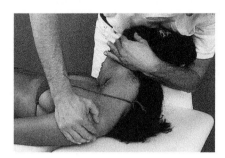

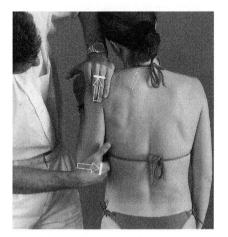

Test of the m. levator scapulae

Stretch and PIR

Anatomy

Origin: Splenius capitis: Spinous processes C7 to T3.

Splenius cervicis: Spinous processes T3 to T6.

Semispinalis capitis: Transverse process C7 to T8 and articular process C3 to C6.

Semispinalis cervicis: Transverse processes T2 to T5.

Course: Splenius: From medial, caudal to lateral, cranial.

Semispinalis: From lateral, caudal to medial, cranial.

Insertion: Splenius capitis: Mastoid process and lateral nuchal line.

Splenius cervicis: Transverse process C1 to C4.

Semispinalis capitis: At the squamous part of the occipital bone next to the midline.

Semispinalis cervicis: Spinous process C2 to C5. Each of the myotenones inserts six to seven vertebral levels above their origin.

Action

With bilateral contraction, extension of the cervical spine and the head. Unilateral contraction rotates and laterally flexes the head and cervical spine to the same side.

Signs of weakness: Bilateral weakness will predispose an anterior head position. Unilateral weakness causes a slight elevation of the occiput on the same side and rotation to the opposite side.

Test

Position: The most simple is to have the patient prone with the arms at the side of the body. The cervical spine is extended first, followed by the head. When testing both sides together, the head must be kept in a neutral position, without rotation. Head rotation of about 45° is made for testing the muscles on one side only.

Stabilization: The free hand is placed beneath, but not touching, the forehead to prevent the nose from crashing into the table surface by a sudden descent of the head when weakness is present.

Test contact: With a broad, non-painful, flat-handed contact to the occiput.

Patient: Pushes the head backwards and upwards as hard as possible.

Examiner: Resists the movement by pushing the back of the head first superiorly, then into flexion by following the arc of motion as it would normally move during flexion/extension.

When testing in a seated or standing position, the examiner must stabilize the patient by placing the one hand on the patient's sternum. The standing position is by far the most demanding with respect to patient stabilization and this must be taken into account. Maintaining the correct resistance direction is of utmost importance because the vector angles change dramatically as the head moves forward on the body.

Test errors, precautions: May be made by any incorrect contact or resistance, by over-stretching the scalp or by compression of the cranial sutures and cervical facets; any of which can lead to false weakness findings. Supporting the body by the elbows during the prone test leads to synergistic recruitment and should be avoided.

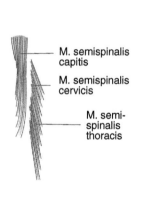

M. semispinalis
capitis

M. semispinalis
cervicis

M. semi-
spinalis
thoracis

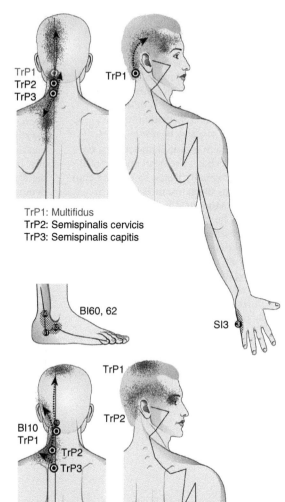

TrP1
TrP2
TrP3

TrP1

TrP1: Multifidus
TrP2: Semispinalis cervicis
TrP3: Semispinalis capitis

Bl60, 62

Sl3

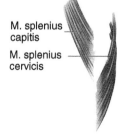

M. splenius
capitis

M. splenius
cervicis

SRS splenius capitis and
cervicis: C7

SRS: According to the '8-rule' the
myotenone, found 8 vertebral
levels above the point of
irritation, will form a myogelosis
Myotenone T8: SRS L4
Myotenone T7: SRS L3, etc.

TrP1

Bl10
TrP1

TrP2

TrP2

TrP3

TrP1: Splenius capitis
TrPs 2 und 3: Splenius cervicis

Bl60, 62

Sl3

Trigger points, referred pain and effective distal points.
In practice, it is difficult to differentiate between the
trigger points due to their close positioning

Myofascial syndrome

Stretch test: An isolated stretch is not possible, as all of the posterior neck extensors (trapezius, levator scapulae and short suboccipital muscles) will be included in the test. When stretch of the muscles on one side only is desired, rotation and lateral inclination to the opposite side can also be used.

PIR: The patient is seated and resting on the back of a chair. The head and cervical spine are maximally flexed so that the chin approximates the sternum. The stretch position is maintained by holding the back of the head down to prevent it from moving up during the procedure. The patient takes and holds an inspiration, then looks up with the eyes while minimally extending the head and neck. The relaxation phase has the patient looking down while breathing out as the examiner gently increases head flexion.

Frequently found associated disorders

A functional weakness of the neck extensors, found when both sides are tested together, may be an indication of micro-fixations of the lumbar spine.

Should one side test weak and the other strong, a micro-fixation of the SI joint on the side of weakness is possible. If both muscles test weak when tested individually, but strong when tested together, a sacral fixation influencing both SI joints is demonstrated.

A hidden cervical disc lesion will often cause dysfunction of individual segments of the neck extensors rather than the entire group.

The neck extensors are always involved as a sequel to whiplash (hyper-extension/flexion) injuries, leading to increased tension and the development of trigger points.

Cause for compression: The greater occipital nerve can be compressed at the level of C4 or C5 by trigger points found within the muscles. Trigger points often develop a few centimetres below the point where the nerve emerges from the semispinalis capitis muscle.

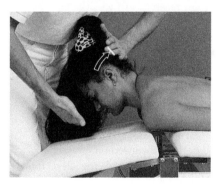

Bilateral neck extensor test

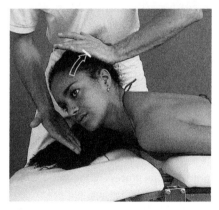

Left neck extensor test

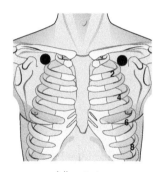

NL anterior

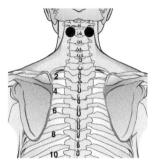

NL posterior

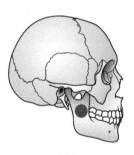

NV

Motor function innervation:
Splenius capitis: C4–C6
Splenius cervicis: C5–C8
Semispinalis capitis: C1–C6
Semispinalis cervicis: C6–C8
Rib pump: Intercostal space, costotransverse joint 3, 4, 8
Meridian: Stomach
Organ: Paranasal sinuses, head lymph system
Nutrients: Vitamins B6 and B3, iodine

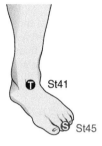

St41

St45

Note: None of the following muscles can be directly or indirectly evaluated using manual muscle testing methods.

M. rectus capitis posterior major

Anatomy

Origin: Spinous process of the axis.

Course: Superiorly, fanning out towards the insertion with the anterior fibres running medially.

Insertion: Lateral half of the inferior nuchal line of the occiput.

Action

One-sided action: Lateral inclination of the head and rotation to the side of the contracting muscle.

Bilateral action: Slight extension of the head made by a rotation of the skull downwards towards the axis.

M. rectus capitis posterior minor

Anatomy

Origin: Tubercle of the posterior arch of atlas.

Course: Below the trapezius and semispinalis capitis.

Insertion: At the medial third of the inferior nuchal line of the occiput. Significantly, there is a deep attachment to the dura mater (Hack et al. 1995).

Action

One-sided action: Lateral inclination of the head.

Bilateral action: Extension of the head by rotating the skull backwards and down towards the posterior arch of atlas. Importantly with respect to craniosacral mechanics, it also tenses the dura mater during contraction.

M. obliquus capitis superior

Anatomy

Origin: Transverse process of C1.

Course: Progresses superior and posteriorly to the insertion.

Insertion: Slightly above the lateral third of the inferior nuchal line.

Action

Unilateral action: Rotation of the head to the opposite side of contraction and aids in lateral inclination to the same side.

Bilateral action: Extension of the head by depressing the occiput towards the atlas and inferior rotation of the occiput.

M. obliquus capitis inferior

Anatomy

Origin: Apex of the spinous process of the axis.

Course: Laterally and slightly superiorly.

Insertion: Transverse process of the atlas.

Action

Rotation of the head to the side of muscle contraction.

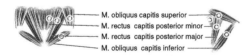

M. obliquus capitis superior
M. rectus capitis posterior minor
M. rectus capitis posterior major
M. obliquus capitis inferior

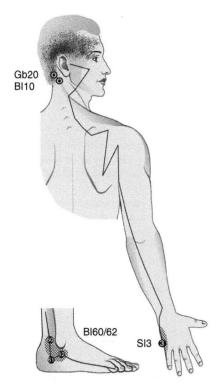

Gb20
Bl10

Bl60/62

Sl3

Trigger points, referred pain and effective distal points

Motor function innervation: Dorsal branches of spinal nerves C1 and C2
Organ: Paranasal sinuses, head lymph system
Nutrients: Vitamins B6 and B3, iodine
SRS:
Rectus capitis posterior major: SI joint
Rectus capitis posterior minor: L5
Obliquus capitis superior: SI joint
Obliquus capitis inferior: SI joint

Anatomy

Origin: Anterior scalene: Anterior tubercle of the transverse processes C2 to C6.

Middle scalene: Posterior tubercle of the transverse processes C2 to C7.

Posterior scalene: Posterior tubercle of the transverse processes C4 to C6.

Longus capitis: Anterior tubercle of the transverse processes C3 to C6.

Longus colli: Vertebral bodies from C5 to T3.

Rectus capitis anterior: Transverse process of the atlas.

Course: All ascend and converge toward the midline of the spine. The middle layers are sandwiched between the sternocleidomastoideus and the upper trapezius muscles. The deeper layer is made up by the longus capitis and longus colli and lies below the prevertebral layer of the neck fascia in direct contact with the vertebral column. The brachial plexus runs through the scalene gap between the scalenus anterior and medius. The omohyoid muscle crosses over the same area, but more superficially, and may irritate the brachial plexus when hypertonic.

Insertion: Anterior scalene: Scalene tubercle at the cranial surface of the 1st rib.

Scalenus medius: Cranial surface of the 1st rib.

Scalenus posterior: Lateral surface of the 2nd rib.

Longus capitis: Interior surface of the basal part of the occiput.

Longus colli: Bodies of C2 to C4.

Rectus capitis anterior: Basal part of the occiput.

Action

The muscles flex the cervical spine and, indirectly, the head. The longus capitis and rectus capitis anterior flex the head directly. With unilateral contraction, the cervical spine laterally flexes and rotates to the opposite side. When the neck is fixed, the scalenus anterior and medius raise the 1st rib and the scalenus posterior raises the 2nd rib. They make up part of the auxiliary respiratory muscles.

Signs of weakness: With weakness on one side, slight rotation of the cervical spine and head to the same side occurs. The patient may have difficulty lifting the head when supine.

Test

Position: The patient is placed supine, the forearms are flexed to 90° and the arms abducted. The arms are then externally rotated and allowed to rest on the table. The arm positioning helps to avoid abdominal recruitment during the test.

The final test position is achieved by flexing the cervical spine, followed by flexion of the head on the neck (in a nodding movement).

The head is held in neutral position for evaluation of both sides simultaneously and rotated 10° to the opposite side for unilateral testing.

Stabilization: The neck flexors can be tested in similar manner with the patient standing or sitting. The examiner uses the free hand to stabilize the upper thoracic spine from behind.

Test contact: A broad contact is made to the patient's forehead with one hand and the free hand is held in a position so as to cushion the head should it abruptly descend when there is pronounced muscle weakness.

Patient: Presses the head upward and forward.

Examiner: Resists by pushing the forehead superiorly and back, following the arc of movement of the head as it flexes from extension.

Test errors, precautions: If the precise resistance vector is not followed, a false weakness may ensue.

Myofascial syndrome

Stretch test (evaluating for adverse tension): The patient is seated on a chair with a sturdy back support. The shoulders are held down by the examiner, followed by extending, then rotating the head to the side opposite the muscle being stretched. The patient can aid in keeping the shoulders down by grasping the seat of the chair and pulling down.

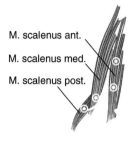

M. scalenus ant.
M. scalenus med.
M. scalenus post.

M. scalenus ant.
M. scalenus med.
M. scalenus post.
M. omohyoideus

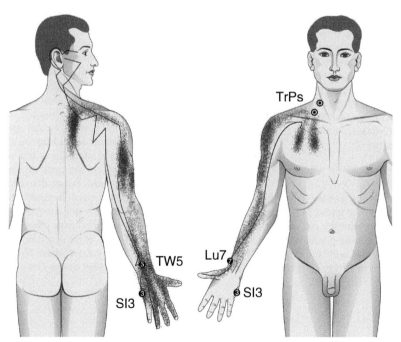

Trigger points, referred pain, and effective distal points of the scalenes

PIR: A deep inspiration is taken and held while the examiner holds the head in the extended position. The patient is asked to first look to the side of the stretched muscle and then look straight down. Then, while slowly breathing out, the patient is instructed to look up and then away from the treated muscle as the examiner gently increases the stretch.

Cause for compression: 'Scalenus syndrome', see below.

Frequently found associated disorders

The neck flexors are adversely affected following almost all whiplash injuries. The resulting trigger points and muscle tension can lead to a scalenus entrapment syndrome with related pain and numbness of the upper extremities.

The neck flexors make up the most proximal site for peripheral compression syndromes of the upper extremities. A number of tests for the diagnosis of scalenus syndrome have been described in the literature – Adson test (Winkel et al. 1985), Scalenus-cramp test (Travell and Simons 1983), Wright test (Winkel et al. 1985) and Eden test (Winkel et al. 1985). Garten (2004) has written a summary of the above tests.

Diagnosis of scalenus syndrome using applied kinesiology

1. The relevant arm muscles innervated by the nerves under investigation are tested with the patient lying in a relaxed, supine position. Most likely the arm muscles will be found to be strong, although in severe cases weakness may be already apparent.

2. With the muscles of the arm found strong in the relaxed position, instruct the patient to lift the head as in the scalenus test. This narrows the gap through which the nerves pass. Rotation of the head towards the arm being examined will tend to layer and overlap the scalenus muscles. Rotation to the opposite side will contract them. If any one of the positions leads to inhibition of the arm muscles, there is a scalenus compression or entrapment.

3. In the same fashion, should the relevant arm muscles already be found weak in the relaxed position, changes in head position may be made in order to provoke a return to strength. Diagnostically, the conclusion will be the same; the only difference being that the point of departure is from weakness rather than strength.

Differential diagnosis for pectoralis minor syndrome

If the arm muscles test 'weak' and none of the head and neck changes described above produce strength, the supine patient's shoulder may be lifted off the table by the examiner. Tension in the pectoralis minor is decreased and constriction of the costoclavicular space reduced. The patient should not be allowed to aid in lifting the shoulder as this will lead to contraction of the pectoralis minor and perhaps increase, rather than reduce tension within the space. In cases where shoulder flexion does not eliminate weakness, the probability of compression at the scalenus gap is indicated or a 'double crush' may exist where both conditions are present at the same time.

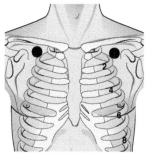

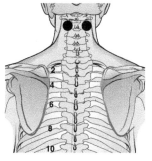

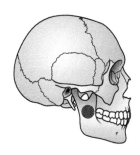

NL anterior

NL posterior

Motor function innervation:
Scalenus anterior: C5–C8
Scalenus medius: C3–C4
Scalenus posterior: C3–C8
Longus capitis: C1–C4
Longus colli: C2–C8
Rib pump: Intercostal space, costotransverse joint 3, 4, 8
Meridian: Stomach
Organ: Paranasal sinuses, head lymph system
Nutrients: Vitamins B6 and B3, iodine
SRS:
Scalene, longus capitis and longus colli muscles: middle thoracic spine

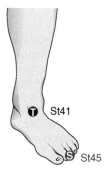

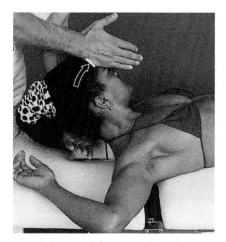

Test of deep neck flexors on the right

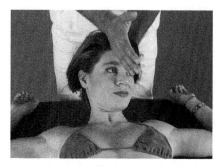

Test of deep neck flexors on the right

Anatomy

Origin: Along the inner aspect of the pelvis that surrounds the obturator foramen and from the obturator membrane.

Course: The muscle forms the anterolateral muscular wall of the lesser (inferior) pelvis. The obturator fascia covers the muscle and is additionally strengthened by an arc of tendons of the levator ani muscles.

Insertion: In the trochanteric fossa.

Action

With the hip in extension, according to Travell and Simons (1992), the internal obturator is predominantly a lateral rotator of the hip, but when the hip is flexed up to 90°, its action is primarily abduction. The muscle regains its function as an external rotator when hip flexion goes beyond 100°. Frick (1992a) notes that the muscle may have an auxiliary capacity in aiding in adduction when the hip joint is in extension.

Test

Position: With the patient supine, the tested leg is allowed to flex naturally at the knee. The thigh is then flexed at the hip to about 110° and laterally rotated so that the foot is moved towards the midline of the body. The other short lateral rotators of the hip are probably all tested as well. The exception to this is the piriformis. In this position it can only abduct and rotate the hip internally.

Test contact: One hand is placed on the lateral aspect of the knee and the other hand on the medial part of the distal leg, close to the internal malleolus.

Patient: In a coupled movement, simultaneously pulls the foot medially and pushes the knee laterally. Most of the emphasis, however, should be made on the medial movement of the foot.

Examiner: Stabilizes the knee to restrict further lateral movement. The main resistance is made by pulling the foot away from the midline.

Test errors, precautions: It is important for proper testing of this muscle that the double action of abduction and lateral rotation of the leg be followed. Regardless as to whether the hip is in extension or in flexion beyond 110° both the external obturator and the quadratus femoris also become adductors. Thus, it is very unlikely that the internal obturator is the only abductor and lateral rotator of the hip during this test. As well, the gemelli muscles cannot be eliminated from the test, either.

As the hip is almost maximally flexed, the piriformis will have no rotatory ability and can be excluded in that at this angle, it can only abduct.

Myofascial syndrome

Stretch test: The maximally flexed thigh is adducted and medially rotated so that the foot moves away from and the knee towards the midline of the body.

PIR: From the stretch position, the patient is instructed to take and hold a deep inspiration for 10 s. The foot is then slowly moved towards the midline of the body which will automatically move the knee away from the midline. The relaxation phase follows by the patient gradually breathing out while the examiner gently brings the foot and knee back to the stretch position and then a bit beyond.

Causes for compression: The adductors and obturatorius externus muscles are innervated by the obturator nerve. Hypertonicity of the obturator muscles may entrap the nerve as it exits the obturator canal and subsequently the adductors weaken.

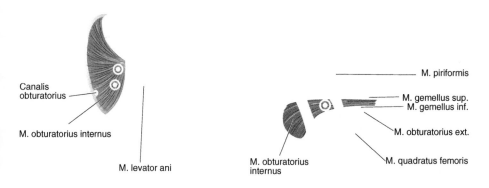

Canalis obturatorius

M. obturatorius internus

M. levator ani

M. piriformis

M. gemellus sup.
M. gemellus inf.

M. obturatorius ext.

M. obturatorius internus

M. quadratus femoris

Motor function innervation: Sacral plexus, L4, L5, S1, (S2)
Visceroparietal segment (TS line): L5
Organ: Gonads
Nutrients: Vitamins A, B3, C, E, PUFA, Zn, Se, Mg
Meridian: Pericardium (circulation)
SRS: T12

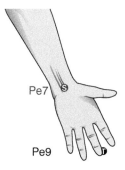

Pe7

Pe9

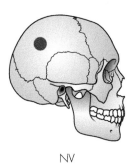

NV

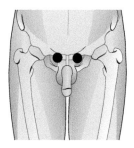

NL anterior

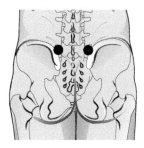

NL posterior

Frequently found associated disorders

Together with the other lateral rotators of the hip (gemelli, obturatorius externus and quadratus femoris), the muscle has special importance as it is in close proximity to the organs of the lesser pelvis. Post-partum tension of the pelvic floor muscles, along with tension in the ligaments anchoring the pelvic viscera, may cause an adverse contraction of the muscle leading to recurrent and chronic hip problems.

Compensatory contraction of the internal obturator muscle as noted above, may cause entrapment of the obturator nerve that, in turn, weakens the adductor muscles causing even greater hip joint imbalance.

Injury to or rupture of the muscle, including fracture of the femoral neck and prosthetic hip replacement, may adversely affect the obturator membrane and lead to dysfunction of other fascial structures of the lesser pelvis. This predisposes a cascade of undesirable, compensatory events that may negatively influence the bladder, uterus and prostate.

A disharmonious relationship between the individual external rotators of the hip may also be noted. An abnormal reciprocal inhibition may be provoked by micro-lesions in the origin or insertions of the various muscles. Vertebral restrictions may also cause weaknesses in one or more of the hip external rotators. As a consequence, strain-counterstrain lesions will be prone to develop in the synergistic muscles.

In the most difficult cases, the mirrored, contralateral muscles may also develop myofascial lesions and reflexively shorten. This is a frequent finding occurring between antagonistic muscle groups.

Compression weakness: Occasionally, the nerve to the obturator internus branches off from the inferior gluteal nerve following its exit from the piriformis and may be compressed in those already suffering from piriformis syndrome.

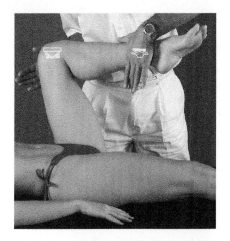

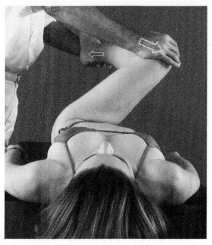

Stretch and PIR with emphasis on the obturatorius internus

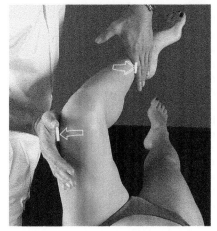

The two illustrations depict the obturator internus test (and other lateral rotators). The 110° hip flexion excludes the piriformis.

M. opponens digiti minimi

Anatomy

Origin: From the hook of the hamate and the flexor retinaculum.

Course: From a more proximal radial area to distal ulnar insertion.

Insertion: The entire length of the ulnar side of the 5th metacarpal bone.

Action

Opposes, flexes, radial abducts and medially rotates the 5th metacarpal bone to oppose it with and move it towards the thenar aspect of the thumb. The combined action of both opponens muscles allows the 'cupping' of the palm.

Signs of weakness: Unable to cup the palm, atrophy of the ball of the little finger.

Test

Position: The little finger is moved so as to oppose the thumb.

Stabilization: In the area of the 1st to 3rd metacarpals on the palmar aspect of the hand and thumb.

Test contact: At the distal aspect of the 5th metacarpal.

Patient: Attempts further movement of the little finger towards the palm and thumb.

Examiner: Actively resists the medial movement by trying to 'open' the palm.

Test errors, precautions: Testing pressure should not be made on the little finger or over the 1st interphalangeal joint.

Myofascial syndrome

Stretch test: Contacting the distal phalanges of the little finger, the 5th metacarpal is abducted and extended. This also stretches the flexor digiti minimi.

PIR: From the stretched position the patient is asked to slowly press in the direction of palmar adduction and opposition. The relaxation phase follows by a gentle return to the start position and then a bit further so that muscle elongation is enhanced.

Cause for compression: Entrapment of the ulnar nerve at the wrist is common following injury to the palm.

Compression weakness: Compression may occur in the ulnar tunnel formed by the pisiform and hamate bones causing ulnar tunnel syndrome; also known as pisiform-hamate syndrome. Due to nerve entrapment at the tunnel the flexor digiti minimi, lumbricals and adductor pollicis muscles will also become functionally weakened.

Compression of ulnar nerve as it passes the elbow (sulcus ulnaris syndrome) will also cause functional opponens digiti minimi weakness. The proximal entrapment will also weaken the flexor carpi ulnaris and flexor digitorum profundus muscles located in the forearm before the wrist.

The muscle can also be used as the indicator muscle for cervical-dorsal junction disc lesions located at C7/T1.

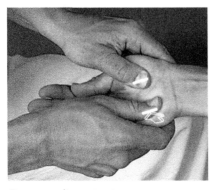
Opponens digiti minimi test

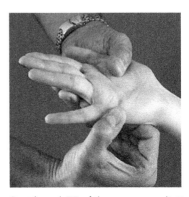
Stretch and PIR of the opponens digiti minimi

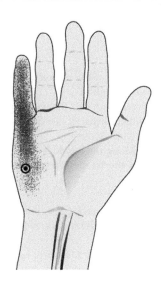

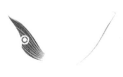

Motor function innervation: Ulnar nerve, C8, T1
Rib pump: Intercostal space, costotransverse joint 10
Nutrients: Ca, Mg, Fe, phosphatase, Vit. B5, PUFA
Meridian: Stomach

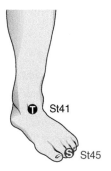

St41

St45

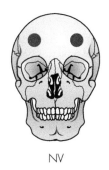

NV

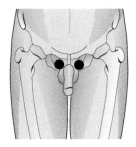

NL anterior

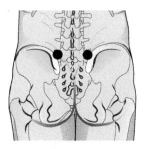

NL posterior

Anatomy

Origin: Tubercle of the trapezium bone and flexor retinaculum.

Course: From medial at the wrist to lateral on the first metacarpal. It lies deep to the abductor pollicis brevis.

Insertion: Along the whole length of the radial side of the 1st metacarpal.

Action

Apposes the 1st metacarpal to the little finger by flexion, palmar adduction, slight rotation.

Signs of weakness: Difficulty holding a pen, weakness when attempting apposition to the little finger. Chronic weakness will cause atrophy, noted by lack of substance at the ball of the thumb.

Test

Position: With all joints of the thumb extended, it is moved towards the little finger.

Stabilization: The lateral aspect of the hand and palm.

Test contact: Head of the 1st metacarpal of the thumb.

Patient: Attempts to move the thumb towards the little finger.

Examiner: Pulls the 1st metacarpal away from the palm in a direction of extension, abduction and lateral rotation.

Test errors, precautions: Test pressure should not be exerted on the thumb itself, but on the head of the 1st metacarpal. Due to the short lever afforded to the examiner, the resistance vector, as described above, must be followed very precisely. During the test, avoid exerting so much resistance pressure that contact pain is elicited. During the test, one should be aware of the synergistic action of the flexor pollicis brevis. Having two heads, one is innervated by the median nerve and the other by the ulnar. The head innervated by the median nerve may be able to compensate for ulnar nerve weaknesses if allowed to enter into the test. Differentiation can be made by testing the adductor pollicis brevis (ulnar nerve) and comparing it to the opponens pollicis (median nerve).

Myofascial syndrome

Stretch test: The thumb is abducted from the palm and extended.

PIR: From the stretch position and while the lateral palm is stabilized by the examiner, the patient is asked to slowly press the thumb in the direction of palmar adduction, flexion and opposition. During the relaxation phase the examiner gently elongates the muscle by bringing the thumb back into the stretched position.

Frequently found associated disorders

With carpal tunnel syndrome a functional weakness of the muscle is evident and, eventually, atrophy occurs.

Cause of compression: Typically carpal tunnel syndrome (see below).

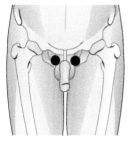

NL anterior

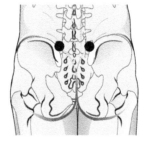

NL posterior

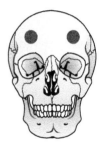

NV

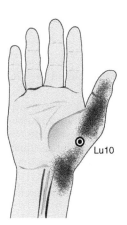

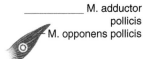

M. adductor pollicis
M. opponens pollicis

Lu10

Motor function innervation: Median nerve, C6, C7
Rib pump: Intercostal space and 10th costotransverse joint
Nutrients: Ca, Mg, Fe, phosphatase, Vitamins B5, PUFA
Meridian: Stomach

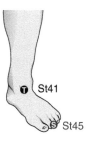

St41

St45

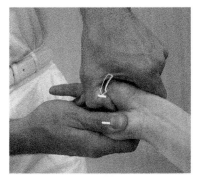

Opponens pollicis test

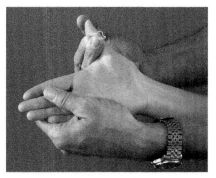

Extension and PIR (tension phase of the opponens pollicis)

M. palmaris longus

Anatomy

Origin: Medial epicondyle of the humerus.

Course: Between the flexor carpi radialis and the flexor carpi ulnaris and on the flexor digitorum superficialis. The tendon runs over the flexor retinaculum.

May be missing in up to 20% of the population.

Insertion: At the palmar aponeurosis of the hand.

Action

Tightens the palmar aponeurosis, helps with palmar flexion in the wrist and cupping the hand.

Test

Position: The patient moulds the hand into a cup and flexes the wrist.

Test contact: With a broad contact on the palm of the hand. The fingers should not be contacted.

Patient: Keeping the fingers together, flexes the hand.

Examiner: Resists attempting to extend the hand on the wrist.

Test errors, precautions: Improper test vector and provoking pain.

Myofascial syndrome

Stretch test: All fingers and metacarpals as well as the wrist are extended.

PIR: Starting from the stretch position, the patient takes and holds an inspiration, while the hand is lightly flexed and moulded into a cup shape. This is followed by the relaxation phase where the stretch position is gently reintroduced while the patient slowly breathes out.

Frequently found associated disorders

The development of Dupuytren's contracture may be associated with trigger points in the palmaris longus even though causality has not been proven (Travell and Simons 1983).

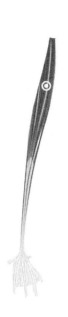

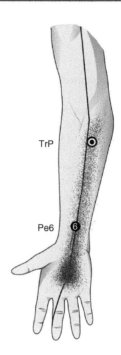

TrP

Pe6

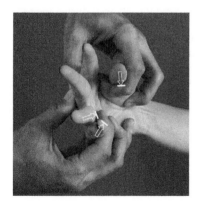

Palmaris longus test

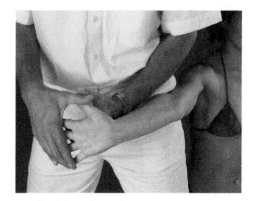

Stretch of the Palmaris longus

Anatomy

Origin: From the medial half of the clavicle.

Course: Progressing from medial to lateral and slightly inferiorly, the fibres merge, crossing over those of the pectoralis sternalis and costalis.

Insertion: At the crest of the greater tubercle of the humerus and lateral margin of the bicipital groove.

Action

Flexion, adduction and medial rotation of the humerus.

Signs of weakness: Retraction of the humerus and scapula. The shoulder may have an increased posterior deviation relative to the body and the opposite shoulder.

Test

Position: From the supine, standing or seated positions, the forearm is internally rotated so that the thumb points down and the arm elevated from the trunk to 90° so that it is perpendicular to the body.

Test contact: Close to the wrist on the dorsal aspect of the distal forearm.

Stabilization: The contralateral shoulder is stabilized. When the test is conducted in the seated or standing position, additional stabilization is made at the shoulder on the side being tested in order to stabilize the trunk and to avoid rotation occuring during testing.

Patient: Keeping the elbow in extension pulls the arm across the chest and slightly upward.

Examiner: Primarily resists in a lateral direction so as to abduct the arm, but also slightly inferiorly (about 15°) to keep the resistance in line with the course of the muscle fibres.

When the muscles on both sides are tested together, stabilization of the contralateral shoulder is not necessary. The examiner contacts the dorsal aspect of both distal forearms and the patient is instructed to pull both extended arms together. Resistance is made simultaneously in a direction of abduction and slight inferiority. Some believe that it is best that the examiner use a 'crossed arms' contact when performing the test, but a short-armed examiner testing a long-armed patient might not be a wise choice.

Test errors, precautions: Allowing the patient to bend the elbow(s) during the test leads to recruitment of the biceps and may falsify findings. The patient should not lift the shoulders nor should the examiner make contact too far distally over the wrist and cover the dorsum of the hand.

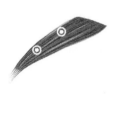

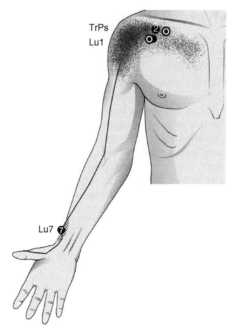

TrPs
Lu1

Lu7

Referred pain and effective distal point

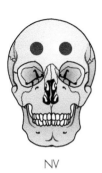

NV

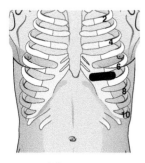

NL anterior

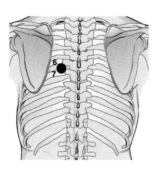

NL posterior

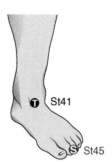

St41

St45

Motor function innervation: Pectoral nerves, C5, C6, C7
Visceroparietal segment (TS line): T5
Rib pump: Intercostal space, costotransverse joint 8, 9
Organ: Stomach
Nutrients: Vitamin B1 (thiamine) with unilateral weakness. Zinc and betaine HCl with bilateral weakness
Meridian: Stomach

Myofascial syndrome

Stretch test: The arm is laterally rotated, abducted to about 60–70° and extended at the shoulder.

PIR: The supine patient, starting with the arm in the stretched position, takes and holds an inspiration for 10 s while lifting the arm without resistance. In the relaxation phase, the patient slowly breathes out while allowing the arm to drop back to the stretch position using only its own weight. The examiner may guide the arm back to the stretched position.

Frequently found associated disorders

Myofascial disorders and trigger points combined with shoulder problems. Bilateral weakness may indicate gastric disorders, usually hypochlorhydria. Goodheart has associated bilateral weakness with a temporal bulge lesion (sidebending) of the cranial vault (Walther 1988).

Cause of compression: Scalenus syndrome, costoclavicular syndrome.

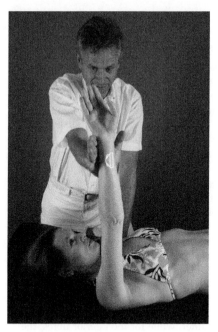

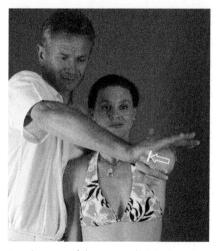

Standing test of the pectoralis major clavicularis. Note: With strong patients, it is recommended to stabilize the trunk from the opposite side and countering the movement with the extended test arm

Pectoralis major clavicularis test

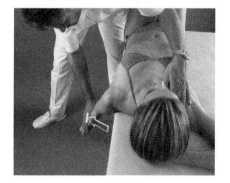

Stretch and PIR in supine position

Anatomy

Origin: From the sternal margin, the cartilage of the 2nd to 7th ribs and the aponeurosis of the obliquus abdominus. The latter two fibre parts are generally differentiated as the pectoralis major costalis and abdominalis. For simplicity, all fibres will be included under the single heading of pectoralis major sternalis.

Course: Converging superiorly and laterally the fibres of the pectoralis major wrap around each other so that the inferior fibres insert to lie under those of the pectoralis clavicularis.

Insertion: Crest of the greater tubercle of the humerus at the lateral margin of the bicipital groove of the humerus. Due to the wrapping effect, the inferior fibres end up having a more superior insertion on the greater tubercle.

Action

With the arm in flexion (as in the test position described below), adduction and medial rotation occur. As well, a slight extension of the humerus can be noted as the more caudal fibres contract. Protraction and depression of the shoulder occur when the arm is fixed.

Signs of weakness: Retraction of the shoulder and scapula. Upon observation, the shoulder will appear further posterior and slightly more superior than in its normal relationship to the trunk.

Test

Position: In the supine, standing or seated position the elbow is extended and with the arm in full medial rotation, it is extended from the trunk to a minimum of 90° and as much as 110° (120° in strong people).

Test contact: On the radial bone of the distal forearm.

Stabilization: For the costal fibres the anterior iliac spine on the opposite side is stabilized, the opposite shoulder when testing the sternal fibres. Testing done in a standing position requires that the patient's trunk be stabilized against rotation by using the free hand, or even the body, if necessary.

Patient: For the superior sternal fibres, the patient pulls the arm towards the opposite shoulder, while for the inferior fibres, the pull is made towards the opposite elbow. The costal fibres are tested by instructing the patient to pull the arm toward the opposite iliac crest.

Examiner: Changes the resistance vector to follow the exact direction for each test.

Test errors, precautions: If the patient is allowed to bend the elbow, the biceps is recruited. The test should not be initiated when it is positioned too far over the body in the direction of the contracted muscle fibre bundle. Without a slight abduction of the arm, the patient may also contract the clavicular division and falsify the test.

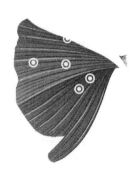

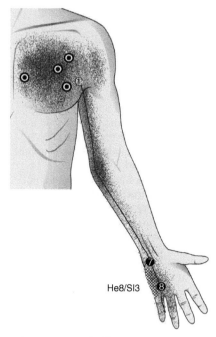

He8/SI3

Referred pain and effective distal points

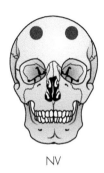

NV

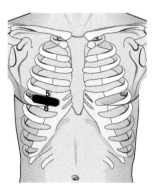

NL anterior

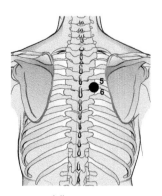

NL posterior

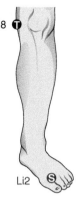

Li8

Li2

Motor function innervation: C6, C7, C8 and T1
Visceroparietal segment (TS line): T8
Rib pump: Intercostal space, costotransverse joint 6
Organ: Liver
Nutrients: Vitamin A, lipotropic factors such as choline, inositol, methionine, vitamin B complex, carduus marianus, bupleurum (Chinese thoroughwax)
Meridian: Liver

Myofascial syndrome

Stretch test: The arm is laterally rotated and abducted so that it moves towards the back, then put in different angles of extension depending upon the fibres to be stretched.

PIR: Is best performed with the patient supine and starting from an extreme stretch position. By changing the arm angles different fibre bundles can be more specifically stretched.

While holding a sustained inspiration, the patient is instructed to bring the arm up against gravity alone. In the relaxation phase, the patient slowly exhales and allows the arm to drop down back to the starting point, again by its own weight. The examiner may increase the stretch very slightly at the endpoint of the natural stretch.

Causes of compression: Lymph vessels originate around the breast tissue and flow into the subclavicular lymph nodes. In the female these can penetrate the pectoralis muscle leading to compression, oedema and increased sensitivity of the breast.

Frequently found associated disorders

Myofascial disorders and trigger point development as a sequel to chronic shoulder dysfunction, causing symptoms of pseudo angina pectoris.

Somatovisceral and viscerosomatic pain reflexes may be caused by trigger points in the right pectoralis major, especially between the 5th and 6th ribs and lead to supraventricular or ventricular extrasystolic arrhythmias (Travell and Simons 1983).

Especially in women with large breasts a shortening of the pectoralis muscles can lead to rounded shoulders and a further shortening of the muscles.

Compression weakness: Can occur with scalenus syndrome and costoclavicular syndrome.

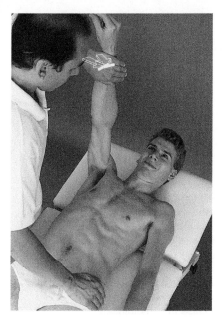

Test of the pectorais major pars costalis. Stabilization of the contralateral pelvis

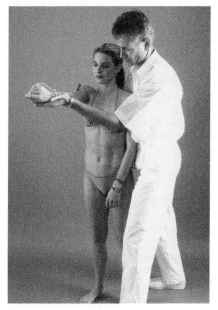

Test of the pectoralis major sternalis in standing position. In very strong patients it is recommended that the examiner stand opposite to the side being tested

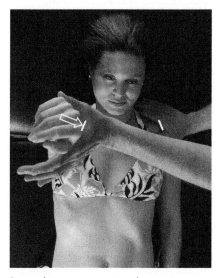

Pectoralis major pars sternalis test

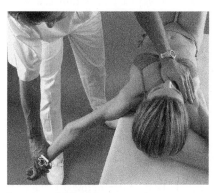

Stretch and PIR of the pectoralis major sternalis. Contraction phase

M. pectoralis minor

Anatomy

Origin: From the 3rd, 4th and 5th ribs near the costocartilagenous junction.

Course: Underlies the pectoralis major muscle. The fibres converge from the ribs in a superior and lateral direction.

Insertion: At the coracoid process of the scapula.

Action

Rotates the scapula anteriorly and protracts the shoulder.

If the insertion on the humerus is the fixed point, it may also act as an auxiliary respiratory muscle by elevating the 3rd to 5th ribs.

Signs of weakness: The shoulder appears to be displaced posteriorly and slightly elevated.

Test

Modified test (Beardall 1993)

Position: The supine patient fully extends the elbow and the arm is put in maximal external rotation. Then the arm is adducted so that the forearm is positioned above the navel and even further in thin, supple patients. Most importantly, the shoulder must be rolled forward so that it lifts from the surface of the table.

Arm rotation should be sufficient to make the palm of the hand point almost anteriorly.

Test contact: On the dorsal aspect of the forearm. The other hand is placed on the anterior shoulder of the side being tested.

Patient: Pulls the forearm towards the navel while attempting to keep the shoulder protracted.

Examiner: Pulls the forearm so as to move it in an arcuate motion away from the abdomen in an anterior–superior direction. At the same time he pushes the shoulder in a superior and posterior direction towards the table surface. The idea is to extend and retract the shoulder by pushing it towards the table surface.

Testing errors, precautions: The examiner must make sure that the humerus is in full external rotation, otherwise synergism from the pectoralis

major sternalis is very pronounced and may invalidate the test.

Kendall (1983) classic test

The patient lies supine and lifts the shoulder from the table surface, protracting the scapula on the thorax.

Contact is made on the anterior aspect of the shoulder with the testing hand and the patient is asked to press the shoulder upward (into protraction) as hard as possible. The examiner resists by pushing the shoulder into retraction.

This test is extremely difficult due to the very short lever and to synergism of the strong pectoralis major sternalis. Thus, it has not proved particularly useful clinically as it does not sufficiently detect functional weakness. Only pronounced weakness in pathologies.

Myofascial syndrome

Stretch test: In the standing position, stretch is made as described in the Wright test (Garten 2012, Winkel et al. 1985), which uses elevation and hyperabduction of the arm to demonstrate coraco-pectoral entrapments of the brachial vascular and nerve bundle.

With the patient supine, the arm is laterally rotated, abducted to 120° and extended. All muscles of the shoulder must be maintained in a relaxed state. This position will retract the scapula on the thorax. Because the arm must be held in lateral rotation, both divisions of the pectoralis major are stretched at the same time.

Signs of shortening: The shoulder is pulled forward and downwards and the arm tends to hang a bit in front of the body.

PIR: With the arm in the stretch position, the patient is asked to breathe in and hold it. While holding the breath, the patient moves the arm and shoulder forward in a direction of flexion and adduction against the examiner's resistance. In the relaxation phase the patient slowly exhales while the examiner gently returns the arm to the stretch position.

Cause for compression: Pectoralis minor syndrome. This most often occurs in people who work with their arms above the head.

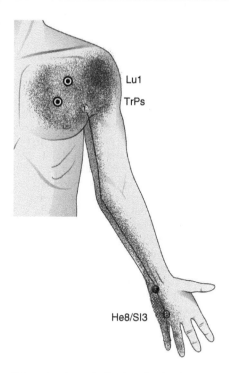

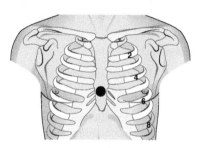

NL reflex

Referred pain and effective distal point

Motor function innervations: Medial pectoral nerve, C6, C7, C8 and T1
Nutrients: Zinc, copper, antioxidants

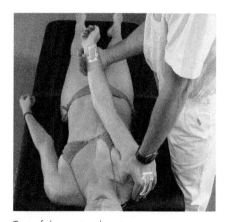

Test of the pectoralis minor

Frequently found associated disorders

Conditions predisposing increased tension and shortening of the muscle are more common that those causing flaccidity. More often than not these are caused by poor posture (hyperkyphosis, juvenile kyphosis and rounding of the shoulders).
Compression weakness: Scalenus syndrome and costoclavicular syndrome.

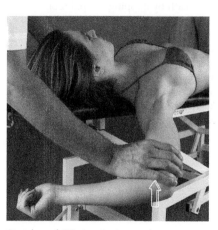

Stretch and PIR: inspiration and contraction

Pelvic floor muscles: M. pubococcygeus

Anatomy

Origin: At the inner surface of the pubic bone.

Course: Runs in a posterior, slightly medial and inferior direction.

Insertion: The medial fibres insert in the central tendon of the perineum and into the fascia of the prostate (prostate levator muscle) in males or the vaginal wall (pubovaginalis) in females.

A bundle of the inferior fibres surrounds the rectum as the puborectalis and form a loop with the contralateral fibres.

The lateral bundle inserts on the coccyx and the sacrum.

Action

It forms a part of the levator ani muscle to lift the pelvic floor and aids in closing the bladder and the rectum. It also helps to stabilize the pelvic organs against ptosis.

Test

Position: The prone patient is instructed to bend the knee at a right angle and lift the leg about 5 to 10 cm above the surface of the table. The femur is then rotated medially to approximately 40° by moving the foot laterally, away from the midline of the body.

Stabilization: On the medial aspect of the opposite knee.

Test contact: The tested leg is supported underneath by cupping the palm of the hand under the knee slightly above the knee cap, so that the 5 cm distance from the table is maintained. The fingers curl upward to contact the medial aspect of the knee.

Patient: Adducts the leg by pulling it towards the other knee as strongly as possible.

Examiner: Resists trying to separate the legs by pulling the knee into abduction.

Note: This action tests an adduction function of the leg. The muscle is not an adductor of the leg as it does not attach to the femur and thus has no direct action on the leg itself. Beardall (1981) was the first to described this test and in practice it appears to have some reliability. An indication of the reliability is concluded as a result of strength changes following treatment of the pubococcygeus muscle. Should the muscle be deemed functional weak, the tested weakness will almost certainly disappear following the application of either an origin-insertion technique (see Ch. 10, Garten 2012) or by stimulating the muscle's lymphatic reflex (see below). Apparently, normal function of the leg adductors is dependent upon the synergism of the pelvic floor muscles.

Test errors, precautions: Functional weakness of the adductors must be ruled out. The examiner should test the adductors for weakness prior to testing the pubococcygeus. Alternatively, the adductors must be tested following a positive test.

Myofascial syndrome

PIR: The muscle cannot be effectively stretched. Nevertheless, Lewit's technique (1992) below may have some therapeutic benefit.

The patient lies in the prone position and grasps the buttocks with both hands, pulling them apart. With gentle resistance and with a sustained inspiration, the patient contracts the buttocks and the pelvic floor as if holding a bowel movement. During the relaxation phase and while breathing out for approximately 10 s, the muscles are allowed to relax while the hands pull the buttocks apart.

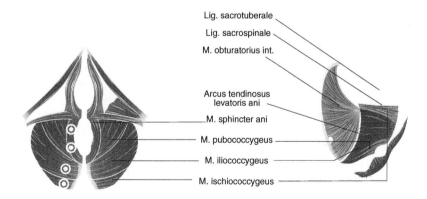

Lig. sacrotuberale
Lig. sacrospinale
M. obturatorius int.

Arcus tendinosus
levatoris ani
M. sphincter ani
M. pubococcygeus
M. iliococcygeus
M. ischiococcygeus

Pelvic floor muscles

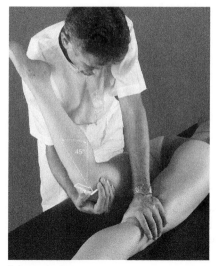

Pubococcygeus test

Motor function innervation: S(4), S5
Meridian: Large intestine
Nutrients: Vitamin E, coenzyme Q10, probiotics (lactobacillus, l-glutamine, etc.)
SRS: Symphysis lesions (caudal sections)

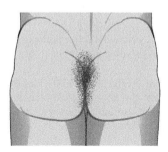

Trigger point and referred pain from the pelvic diaphragm

Frequently found associated disorders

Noted in cases of coccydynia and in women experiencing pain during sexual intercourse, especially during initial penetration. In men, pain in the area of the perineum during ejaculation is symptomatic.

Any post-partum symptom related to the pelvic floor, with or without an episiotomy and symptoms of incontinence whereby the individual has a sense of urgency for evacuation. Prolapsed abdominal organs and pelvic lesions are common, as well. All muscles that traverse the body along the transverse plane, including the pelvic, upper and middle thoracic diaphragms, should be regarded and treated as a unit.

M. iliococcygeus

Anatomy

Origin: At the inner surface of the pubic bone or the ischium as far as the ischial spine, at the tendinous arch of the levator ani muscle.

Course: Lying behind the pubococcygeus muscle, it progresses anterior to posterior and medial.

Insertion: At the lateral margin of the coccyx and the anococcygeum ligament made up of a tough fibrous tract between the anus and the coccyx.

Action

Lifts the pelvic floor and supports the pelvic organs.

Test

Position: The prone patient is instructed to bend the leg at knee and lift it about 10 cm from the surface of the table. There is no rotation of the femur.

Stabilization: The medial aspect of the contralateral leg at the level of the knee passing over the tested leg to grasp the leg from the behind.

Test contact: The tested leg is supported by one hand placed below the knee just above the kneecap and the fingers are curled around and upward to contact its medial aspect.

Patient: Pulls the knee in adduction towards the other leg.

Examiner: Resists in abduction by pulling laterally attempting to separate the legs.

Test errors, precautions: As described for the pubococcygeus muscle.

Myofascial syndrome

PIR: See above m. pubococcygeus.

M. coccygeus (also m. ischiococcygeus)

Anatomy

Origin: Medial surface of the ischial spine.

Insertion: On the anterior surface of the distal sacrum and the coccyx.

Action

The muscle often has more tendinous than contractile fibres and merges into and supports the sacrotuberal ligament.

Test

Position: The prone patient is instructed to bend the lower leg to 90° and laterally rotate the femur about 45° by moving the foot towards the midline of the body.

Stabilization: On the contralateral leg at the level of the knee.

Test contact: With the hand placed to support the leg from below, just above to the kneecap.

Patient: Pulls the knee into adduction towards the other leg.

Examiner: Resists by pulling the leg laterally into abduction.

Test errors, precautions: As described for the pubococcygeus muscle.

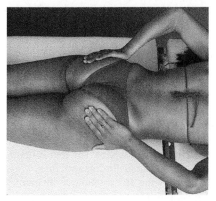

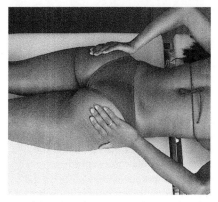

PIR of the gluteal muscles and the pelvic floor: contraction phase with sustained inspiration

PIR of the gluteal muscles and the pelvic floor: relaxation phase with slow expiration

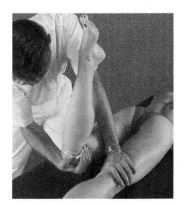

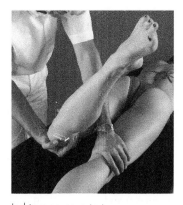

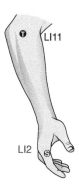

Iliococcygeus test

Ischiococcygeus test

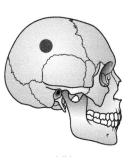

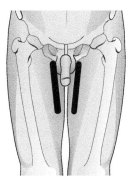

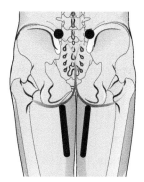

NV

NL anterior

NL posterior

Mm. peronei (brevis and longus)

Anatomy

Origin: Peroneus longus: From the lateral part of the tibial condyle, the head and proximal two-thirds of the lateral surface of the fibula, intermuscular septum and deep fascia of the leg.

Peroneus brevis: Distal two-thirds of the lateral surface of the fibula and the bordering intermuscular septum.

Course: The peroneus brevis lies on the fibula for its entire length and is deep to the more superficial peroneus longus. Two intermuscular septa separate them from the surrounding muscles. One septum is more anterior and overlies the extensor digitorum and tibialis anterior muscles, while the other is more posterior, overlying the soleus and the gastrocnemius muscles.

Insertion: Peroneus longus: Its long tendon passes behind the lateral malleolus, curving under the lateral side of the foot to insert into the lateral side of the base of the 1st metatarsal and the medial cuneiform bone.

Peroneus brevis: Tuberosity of the 5th metatarsal.

Action

The both act to pronate (evert) and plantar flex the foot. They also assist in maintaining lateral balance of the body as well as stabilization of the foot during walking. Travell states that they are primarily active during the push-off phase when walking. But they are mainly for fine foot control rather than used for propulsion of the leg from the ground. (Travell and Simons 1992).

Signs of weakness: Inversion of the foot when walking.

Test

Position: Test of the left peroneus longus and brevis.

The patient is supine and the examiner stands at the foot end of the table. The right hand grasps the patient's forefoot so that the thumb is on the dorsum of the foot and the fingers on the plantar aspect. Contact is made by the thumb web at a point on the distal, lateral part of the 5th metatarsal bone, just below the metatarsophalangeal joint. The foot is first brought into plantar flexion and, then, without allowing any rotation of the foot and tibia, put into abduction and pronation.

As an alternative to the above, the examiner stands/sits on the side opposite to the foot being tested. (Note: It may be necessary to bend the non-tested leg so that the foot is moved away from the testing area.) The palm of the hand is placed so that it covers the plantar aspect of the foot while the thumb lies on the dorsum and the fingers curl around the 5th metatarsal bone. As with the first test, the foot is placed in maximum plantar flexion, abduction and pronation.

Test contact: On the distal, lateral aspect of the 5th metatarsal.

Stabilization: The right hand is placed under the heel to stabilize the calcaneus.

Patient: Keeping the foot in plantar flexion, attempts to abduct the foot as hard as possible.

Examiner: Resists primarily attempting to adduct, but also pulling the foot slighty into dorsiflexion.

The examiner's hand position is reversed in both tests for the right peroneus longus and brevis test.

Test errors, precautions: The testing vectors must be very precise. Due to the short lever and very strong synergism of the foot muscles, any leg rotation or dorsiflexion (extension) of the foot will tend to negate any positive findings. During the test, pain on any of the contact sites should be avoided.

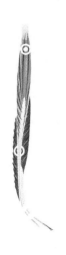

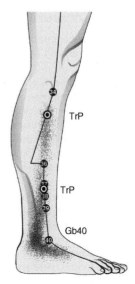

TrP

TrP

Gb40

Referred pain and effective
local and distal points

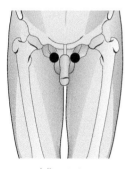

NL anterior

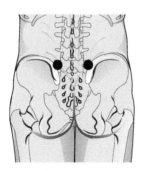

NL posterior

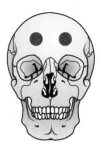

Bl65 Bl67

Motor function innervation: Superficial fibular nerve, L4, L5, S1
Rib pump: Intercostal space, costotransverse joint 3, 4, 8, 9
Organ: Bladder
Nutrients: Vitamin A, vitamin B complex with emphasis on the B1
components, potassium
Meridian: Bladder
SRS: L5

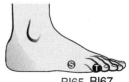

NV

Myofascial syndrome

Stretch test: The foot is put into dorsiflexion (extension) and supination (inversion).

PIR: From the above stretch position, the patient, during a time span of 7–10 s, slowly presses the foot into plantar flexion and eversion. Thereafter, the examiner gently brings the foot back to the starting position and then a bit more. Because the muscle is so distal, no breathing pattern is necessary.

Cause for compression: Entrapment at the peroneal tunnel. Both the superficial peroneal nerve to the peroneus longus and brevis, and the deep peroneal nerve to the tibialis anterior, extensor digitorum longus, extensor hallucis longus, peroneus tertius and extensor digitorum brevis, arch around a point just distal to the head of the fibula and the tendon of the peroneus longus. Increased tension and shortening of the peroneus longus may irritate both nerves leading to dysfunction of all of the above muscles, as well as symptoms of paresthesia on the dorsum of the foot between the 1st and 2nd metatarsals.

Frequently found associated disorders

Lateral instability of the ankle with a tendency to supination trauma is most often noted. Weakness of both the muscles may be associated with injuries to the tibiofibular syndesmosis where the tibia and fibula have been subject to separation trauma. Should this be the case, a manual approximation of the syndesmosis will tend to strengthen the muscles.

Compression weakness: Iliolumbar ligament syndrome, piriformis syndrome, and peroneal tunnel syndrome as noted above.

Lesion of the S1 root, from the L5/S1 disc, leads to weakness of both muscles. (Patten 1998, Walther 2000).

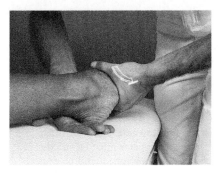

Peroneus brevis and longus test

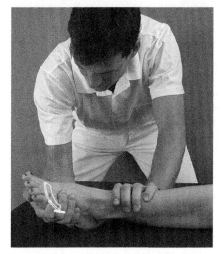

Alternative test position for peroneus brevis and longus

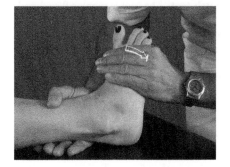

Stretch and PIR of the peroneus longus and brevis: contraction phase

Anatomy

Origin: Distal third of the anterior surface of the fibula, interosseous membrane and bordering intermuscular septum.

Course: Can be regarded as part of the extensor digitorum longus. It lies in the anterior muscle compartment and its tendon runs anteriorly to the external malleolus like those of the other dorsal extensors.

Insertion: Dorsal surface of the base of the 5th metatarsal.

Action

Pronation and dorsal extension of the foot. When walking it stabilizes the foot laterally following heel lift.

Signs of weakness: Drop foot tendency with inversion when walking.

Test

Position: The examiner sits or stands at the foot of the table to make it easy to grasp the patient's foot.

Test contact (left foot): Using the palm and thenar aspects of the right hand, the examiner takes a broad contact on the lateral part of the dorsum of the foot. The fingers wrap around to grasp the plantar side of the foot while a pisiform contact is made just proximal the little toe.

Stabilization: The free hand, medial to the foot, cups and holds the heel of the foot.

Patient: Pulls the lateral aspect of the foot up, into dorsal extension as hard as possible.

Examiner: Resists by pushing the distal, lateral foot into plantar flexion and from slightly lateral to medial direction.

Hand positioning is reversed for the right peroneus tertius.

Testing errors, precautions: The foot must not be allowed to move or rotate and the precise test vector must be strictly followed. Also no pain should be caused by either the testing or stabilizing hands.

Myofascial syndrome

Stretch test: The foot is plantar flexed and inverted (supinated).

PIR: Starting from the above stretch position, and while holding a deep inspiration for about 10 s, the patient gently pulls the foot upward into dorsal extension and eversion (pronation). The patient is then instructed to breathe out while the examiner slowly brings the foot back to a point slightly beyond the start position in order to slightly exaggerate the muscle stretch.

Frequently found associated disorders

Lateral ankle instability. Weakness of the muscle has been noted when there is a concomitant lateral lesion of the cuboid.

A sustained digital pressure (medial challenge) may be made on the cuboid while testing the muscle. The adverse relationship between the two is confirmed when the manoeuvre eliminates the weakness.

Compression weaknesses: L5 or S1 root, iliolumbar ligament, piriformis and fibular tunnel syndromes.

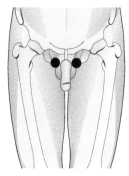

NL anterior

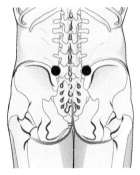

NL posterior

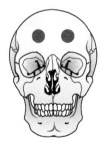

NV

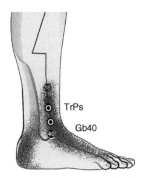

Referred pain pattern, local
and distal points

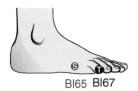

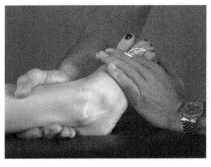

Bl65 **Bl67**

Motor function innervation:
Superficial fibular nerve, L5, S1
Rib pump: Intercostal spaces and
costotransverse joints of the 3rd, 4th,
8th and 9th costal areas.
Organ: Bladder
Nutrients: Vitamin A, B-complex group
with an emphasis on thiamin (B1),
potassium
Meridian: Bladder
SRS: L1, L3

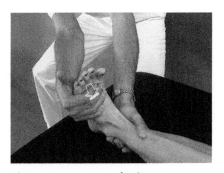

Stretch and PIR of the peroneus tertius:
contraction phase

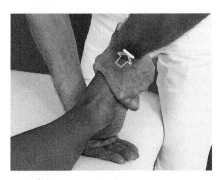

Test of the peroneus tertius

Alternative test position for the peroneus tertius

Anatomy

Origin: From the anterior surface of the sacrum (1st to 4th sacral segment), the capsule of the SI joint and the sacrospinous ligament.

Course: From a broad origin on the sacrum in a lateral direction passing through the sciatic foramen to the greater trochanter.

Insertion: On the posterolateral, superior surface of the greater trochanter.

Action

When the leg is in a straight plane with the body lateral (external) rotation of the femur is most prominent. If the leg is fixed against rotation, it aids in its abduction. As the hip is flexed the muscle becomes an abductor of the leg. With hip flexion beyond 110°, it becomes a medial rotator (Travell and Simons 1992).

According to Travell and Simons (1992) the piriformis is essentially a lateral rotator, especially with the leg in extension, and at 90° flexion, according to Frick et al. (1992), predominately an abductor. Frick also notes that when standing the piriformis also has an auxiliary function of leg abduction. The piriformis is a powerful stabilizer of the iliosacral joint and it prevents the femur from rotating medially when walking. Like the rotary cuff muscles of the shoulder, it helps to fixate the head of the femur in the acetabulum. It also contributes in the early phase of extension of the leg.

Signs of weakness: Medial rotation of the femur, especially seen during the swing phase of the gait.

Test

Classic test in the prone position (Kendall and Kendall 1983)

The prone position primarily tests the ability of the piriformis to externally rotate the femur. The other short lateral rotators of the hip, from which the piriformis cannot be isolated, are tested at the same time.

Position: The knee is flexed to 90° and the femur is abducted to about 30° and externally rotated (the patient's foot moves towards the midline).

Stabilization: The hand stabilizes the lateral aspect of the knee.

Test contact: The testing hand contacts the lower leg close to the medial malleolus.

Patient: Presses the foot medially into the examiner's hand.

Examiner: Resistance by the examiner is from medial to lateral on the distal lower leg attempting to bring the foot away from the midline.

Coupled movement in the supine position

This tests the combined movements of lateral rotation and abduction when the leg is in intermediate flexion.

Note: 'Intermediate flexion' is defined as being about 45–70° of hip flexion (the specific position is somewhat fluid) as measured from the resting position on the table surface. This test is thought to be more precise as it evaluates the dual action of the muscle more specifically and helps to eliminate synergism from the other external rotators.

Position: In the supine position, the femur is flexed less than 90° and with about 30–45° abduction. As in the prone test, the knee is flexed to 90°.

Test contact: One hand laterally at the knee, the other hand medially to the distal lower leg.

Stabilization: There is no real stabilization hand in this test as both are used to resist the combined movement of the patient. Both are stabilizers and both are movers (s. above).

Patient: In a coupled movement, presses the knee laterally into abduction against the one hand and the foot medially into the other hand. Movement into abduction should be the main tested component.

Examiner: Examiner resistance should concentrate more on the adduction of the knee than rotation of the femur. The counter-pressure against the medial

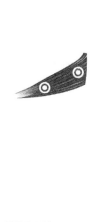

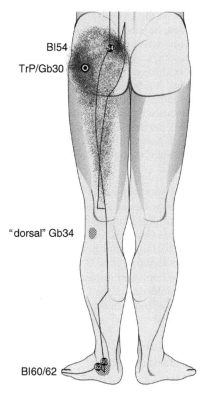

BI54

TrP/Gb30

"dorsal" Gb34

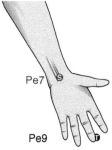

Pe7

Pe9

BI60/62

Referred pain and effective distal points

Motor function innervation: Sacral plexus, L5, S1, S2
Visceroparietal segment (TS line): L5
Organ: Gonads
Nutrients: Vitamins A, B3, C, E, PUFA, Zn, Se, Mg
Meridian: Pericardium (Circulation-Sex)
SRS: L5

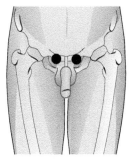

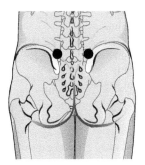

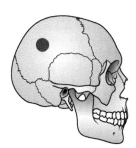

NL anterior   NL posterior   NV

movement on the lower leg is just a stabilization, because otherwise the other external rotators of the hip are tested. Muscle testing accuracy will improve if a dry run or 'dress rehearsal' is made prior to the actual test being performed. Due to the complicated double movement pattern, some patients will benefit by rehearsing the movements one or even two times. With muscle testing, the best maxim is; 'when in doubt, repeat, and repeat again until satisfied'.

Test in the seated position

The position of the leg is identical to that in the supine position in that the hip and knee are flexed up to 90°. It is important to make sure that the femur is abducted about 30° and not flexed beyond 90° at the hip.

The most important movement during the test is abduction of the knee. Greater care should be made in stabilizing the patient against rotation of the body during the test.

Test contact: With the testing hand from medial to distal lower leg.

Stabilization: The free hand stabilizes the lateral knee.

Patient: Presses the foot in a medially and the knee laterally into the examiners hands as firmly as possible.

Test errors, precautions: The most important factor distinguishing the piriformis from the other external rotators is that it has no external rotatory capacity when the hip is in flexion. During the test, the rotatory component by the examiner should be minimized, or the test may favour the other external rotators rather than the pirifomis. In the supine position, the femur must not be flexed more than 60–70° as the piriformis becomes a medial rotator with about 110° of hip flexion. Rotation of the pelvis by the patient should be restricted.

Myofascial syndrome

Stretch test: In prone position the knee is flexed to 90° and the femur medially rotated (the foot and lower leg are moved laterally) to its natural endpoint.

The test can also be performed in the supine position. The femur is flexed to 90°.

The examiner presses the knee and femur towards the table (posteriorly) and adducts the thigh while maintaining posterior pressure at the knee. This prevents lifting of the pelvis during the test. At the same time, the lower leg and foot are moved laterally which imposes a medial rotation of the femur and additional stretch of the piriformis.

PIR: Starting from the stretch position the patient is instructed to slowly contract the piriformis by pushing the foot and lower leg medially and the knee laterally. A sustained inspiration is held by the patient during the muscle contraction. As the patient breathes out, the leg is gently brought back to the stretch position and then slightly more to pronounce the stretch effect. The therapeutic contraction and elongation directions are the same for both supine and prone positions.

Causes for compression: Muscle tension can lead to compression in the area of the sciatic foramen. The superior and inferior gluteal nerves, the sciatic nerve and the pudendal nerve may be affected. This can lead to weakness of the gluteus maximus, the gluteus medius, gluteus minimus and the tensor fasciae lata. In addition, the hamstrings, anterior and posterior tibalis, entire superficial and deep fibular group and intrinsic foot muscles will be affected.

A chronic weakness of the gluteus maximus may lead to an increased contraction of the piriformis on the same side. The resulting cascade of weakness, entrapment, lower limb weakness and gait disturbance can lead to a vicious cycle of perpetual dysfunction.

Frequently found associated disorders

Imbalance of the piriformis always occurs with a category 1 pelvic lesion (according to sacro-occipital technique (SOT) by DeJarnette). Bilateral functional weakness is most often indicative of disorders of the organs of the lesser pelvis.

Hypertonus and contraction of the piriformis can lead to irritation of the sciatic nerve (piriformis syndrome). Some describe a condition in which the piriformis is unduely stretched as the cause of the syndrome. The literature, however, is not clear on the subject. Therefore, orthopaedic tests vary from stretching to contraction of the piriformis in order to provoke pain. As well, the literature vacillates from describing it as a rare occurring phenomenon to one of hidden frequency. This is probably due to the fact that there is no real accord as to where, when and how it is diagnosed. AK testing adds another dimension to this diagnostic process. Nevertheless, in both cases the syndrome is frequently confused with lumbar disc problems. More often than not the syndrome is a sequel to lumbar disc problems. Compression of the gluteal and pudendal nerves can also occur (see above).

Causes of compression: S1 root syndrome from the L5/S1 intervertebral foramen and iliolumbar ligament syndrome. With the iliolumbar ligament syndrome, the L5 root is irritated as it passes through the lumbosacral tunnel.

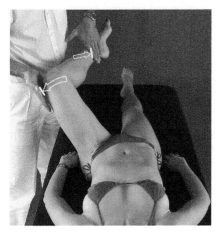

Test of piriformis in supine position

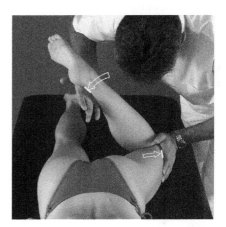

Test of piriformis in prone position

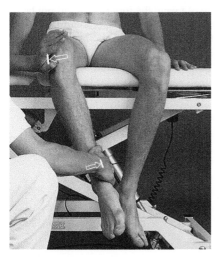

Test of piriformis in seated position

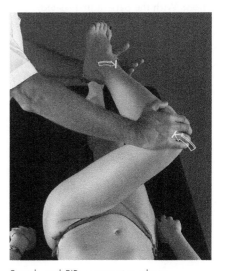

Stretch and PIR: contraction phase

Anatomy

Origin: Arises from the distal part lateral epicondyle of the femur, the posterior capsule of the knee, the lateral meniscus and (in some texts) the fibular head.

Course: The tendon of the origin runs from the lateral condyle of the femur superficial to the articular capsule and underneath the lateral collateral ligament. The muscle fans out medially and distally from the insertion.

Insertion: Posterior surface of the tibia on the upper half of the soleal line.

Action

With the femur fixed, the tibia is medially rotated. When standing and with the lower leg fixed, it laterally rotates the thigh. It functions as a knee flexor and pulls the knee out of pronounced hyperextension when standing as well as stabilizing the lateral aspect of the knee. When the knee is bent it pulls the lateral meniscus posteriorly. During heel strike of the gait cycle, the muscle helps to stabilize the knee and absorption of the force of impact.

Signs of weakness: Hyperextension of the knee.

Test

Position: With the patient in a seated, supine or prone position, the knee is flexed to 90° and maximally internally rotated so that the toes of the foot move toward the midline. As well, the foot is maintained in neutral position with regard to flexion/extension and inverted so the ankle joint is locked down.

Test contact: On the medial aspect of the patient's forefoot, close to the great toe.

Stabilization: On a large area covering the lateral calcaneus and lateral malleolus.

Patient: Presses the forefoot into medial rotation as firmly as possible.

Examiner: Resists in the direction of lateral rotation. The popliteus is considered to be weak if the foot moves away from the midline and the tibial tuberosity is seen to rotate laterally during the test. The lateral rotation of the tibial tuberosity is the determining factor. However, if the foot does not move, neither does the tibial tuberosity and the muscle may be considered strong.

If the movement of the tibial tuberosity is not noted, yet the foot everts and rotates laterally during the test, there is lack of stabilization of the foot at the ankle and the popliteus test cannot be made until corrected. The anterior and posterior tibialis muscles must then be tested before further evaluation of the popliteus may be made.

Test errors, precautions: When there is a lack of ankle stability a differential test of the tibialis muscles must be made. Avoid causing pain in the area of the heel or the ankle. As well, the forefoot should not be too tightly gripped by the examiner contact as this can lead to pain and false weakness findings.

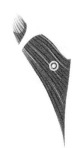

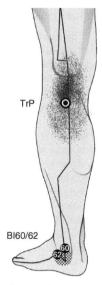

TrP

Bl60/62

Effective distal points

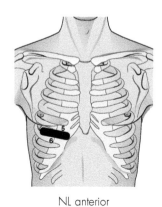

NL anterior

NL posterior

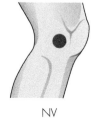

NV

Motor function innervation: Tibial nerve, L4, L5, S1
Visceroparietal segment (TS line): T4
Rib pump: Intercostal space, costotransverse joint 4
Organ: Gallbladder
Meridian: Gallbladder
Nutrients: Vitamin A, essential fatty acids (PUFA)
SRS: L4

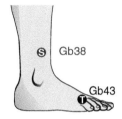

Gb38

Gb43

Myofascial syndrome

Stretch test: In the supine position the knee is extended and the heel of the patient is lifted from the table. The lower leg is then laterally rotated as far as possible. This will maximize lateral rotation of both the knee and hip joints.

The level of lateral rotation in the hip joint can be compared with the overall lateral rotation if the knee joint. The degree of rotation of the leg at the knee, as opposed to that of the hip, may be made by bending the knee to 90° and repeating the lateral rotation of the lower leg. Thus, determining the actual degree of lateral rotation at the hip joint is made much easier.

PIR: Starting from the stretch position, the lower leg is slowly rotated medially while the patient holds a sustained inspiration. As the patient breathes out, and without any resistance, the examiner rotates the leg laterally to bring it back to the stretch position. Slightly more rotation is induced at the natural endpoint of movement to further enhance the stretch.

Frequently found associated disorders

Chronic knee instability and difficulty in rehabilitation following knee surgery.

Cause of compression: L5 root syndrome from the L4/L5 intervertebral foramen, piriformis syndrome, iliolumbar ligament syndrome.

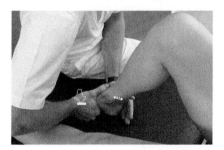

Popliteus test in the supine position

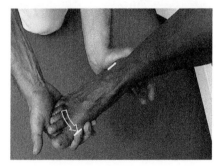

Popliteus test in the seated position

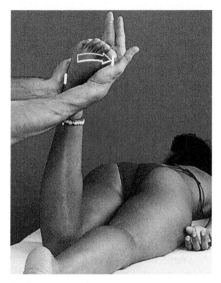

Popliteus test in the prone position

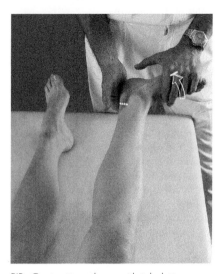

PIR: Contraction phase with inhalation.

M. pronator quadratus

Anatomy

Origin: Distal quarter of the ulnar and palmar surface of the ulna.

Course: Progressing from medial to lateral in the deepest muscle layer of the palmar side of the forearm.

Insertion: Distal quarter of the radial and palmar surface of the radius.

Action

Together with the pronator teres it pronates of the forearm.

Signs of weakness: An increased supination may be seen at the hand when the arm is in a relaxed, hanging position.

Test

Position: The forearm is fully flexed at the elbow and then pronated.

Test contact: With one hand on the distal forearm. The distal forearm affords a very weak contact for resistance. As some significant strength must be used, it can be an advantage if the examiner encircles the distal forearm and fist with both hands and folds the fingers, providing a broad, strong testing pressure that is not so profound as to cause pain. A broad contact by wrapping both hands around the patient's fist may be advisable in strong patients. Care must be taken not to contact certain acupuncture points in the area.

Stabilization: If not using both hands for resistance, the free hand stabilizes the humerus in the area of the elbow.

Patient: Pronates the forearm as much as possible.

Examiner: Resists by trying to supinate the wrist and forearm.

Test errors, precautions: Pain caused by hand contacts. It is impossible to fully eliminate the synergistic effect of the pronator teres.

Myofascial syndrome

Stretch test, PIR: Is made together with the pronator teres.

Frequently found associated disorders

Muscle weakness that leads to an abnormal lengthening of the flexor retinaculum can cause medial nerve entrapment and carpal tunnel syndrome. Therapy consists of local origin-insertion treatment (see Ch. 10, Garten 2012).

Causes for compression: Carpal tunnel syndrome.

Compression weakness

Pronator teres syndrome whereby the median nerve is entrapped as it passes between the ulnar and radial head of the pronator teres. Diagnosis is confirmed by a weakness pattern demonstrated in other muscles found distal to the pronator teres. These would include the flexor pollicis longus, flexor digitorum profundus (2nd and 3rd fingers), flexor pollicis longus, pronator quadratus and the muscles of the ball of the thumb, with the exception of the adductor pollicis and the deep head of the flexor pollicis brevis.

A C8 root syndrome from the C7/T1 intervertebral foramen. Disturbances caused by a more proximal entrapment, like scalenus, costoclavicular and pectoralis minor syndromes as well as the median nerve at the axilla may all cause weakness of the pronator quadratus.

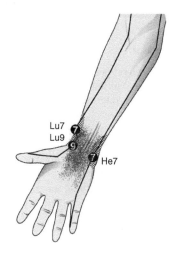

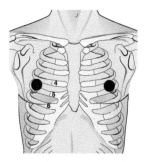

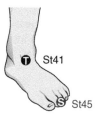

Motor function innervation: Median nerve, C7, C8, T1
Organ: Stomach
Meridian: Stomach
Nutrients: Ca, Mg, Fe, phosphatase (e.g. from raw potatoes), vitamin B5, PUFA

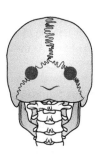

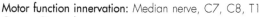

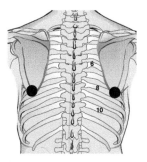

NL anterior   NL posterior   NV

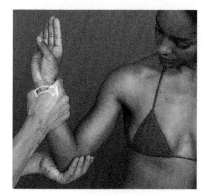

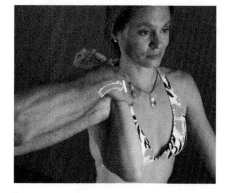

Pronator quadratus test

Anatomy

Origin: Humeral head: Arises from the anterior surface of the medial epicondyle of the humerus, intermuscular septum and antebrachial fascia.

Ulnar head: Medial surface of the coronoid process of the ulna.

Course: Found in the same layer as, but more lateral, to the flexor carpi radialis.

Insertion: In the middle of the ulnar surface of the radius.

Action

With the pronator quadratus, pronation, and some auxiliary flexion, of the forearm.

Signs of weakness: When the arm is left to hang down, an increased supination of the hand may be seen.

Test

Position: The forearm is flexed by 45° and fully pronated.

Test contact: To the distal part of the patient's forearm or fisted hand with no flexion/extension of the wrist.

Stabilization: At the elbow if not using both hands.

Patient: Strongly pronates the forearm.

Examiner: Supination of the forearm.

Test errors, precautions: The testing hand contact must not be painful. A two-hand contact can be made more firmly without causing pain.

A common compensation for weakness is to abduct the elbow from the trunk during the test. Restricting this tendency is essential.

Myofascial syndrome

Stretch test: The forearm is supinated and the elbow extended. Muscle shortening is common and stretching may activate latent trigger points, leading to referred pain.

PIR: The patient rotates the forearm from the stretch position into pronation against the examiners resistance. In the relaxation phase, the therapist gently stretches into supination and slightly beyond.

Causes for compression: Pronator teres syndrome leads to irritation of the median nerve as described for the pronator quadratus. Diagnosis is confirmed by weakness of the muscles distal to the pronator teres: flexor pollicis longus, flexor digitorum profundus (2nd and 3rd fingers), flexor pollicis longus, pronator quadratus and the muscles of the ball of the thumb. Muscles like the adductor and deep head of the flexor policis, having ulnar innervation, are exceptions.

The pronator teres syndrome can eventually also lead to double crush of the median nerve by provoking a carpel tunnel syndrome due to the subsequent inhibition of the pronator quadratus.

Frequently found associated disorders

Compression weakness: C7 root symptoms arising from the intervertebral foramen of C6/C7, scalenus syndrome, costoclavicular syndrome and pectoralis minor syndrome.

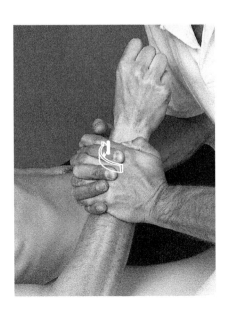

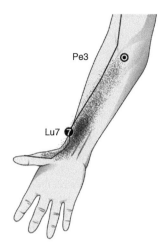

Pe3

Lu7

Motor function innervation: Median nerve, C6, C7
Organ: Stomach
Meridian: Stomach
Nutrients: Ca, Mg, Fe, Phosphatase, PUFA, Vitamin B5

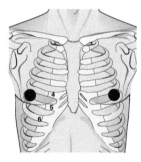

NL anterior

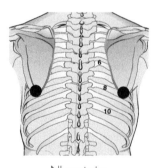

NL posterior

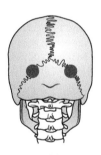

NV

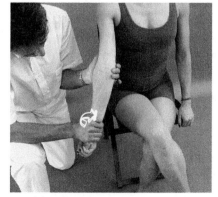

PIR of the pronator teres

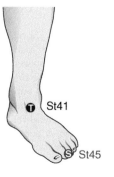

St41

St45

Anatomy

Origin: From the vertebral bodies and intervertebral discs of T12 to L5, as well as from the transverse processes L1 to L5.

Course: Progresses from superior to inferior and slightly anterior and lateral. The psoas and iliacus form the dorsal muscular cushion for the kidneys and provide the fascial surface for the attachment of the caecum on the right and the sigmoid colon on the left.

Insertion: In a common insertion with the iliacus on the posteromedial aspect of the lesser trochanter.

Action

Flexion and adduction of the femur and, with the hips in a neutral position, a slight medial rotation is possible (Palastanga et al. 1989, Schiebler et al. 1999). When the hip is flexed and abducted, a slight lateral rotation component is evident (Walther 2000, Kendall and Kendall 1983, Travell and Simons 1992). This is due to the fact that the insertion angle changes with respect to the pivot point (see also iliacus muscle).

In the standing position and with the thigh as a fixed point, a simultaneous contraction of both sides will rotate the pelvis posteriorly and lordose the lumbar spine. One-sided contraction will tip the ilium posteriorly, side-bend the lumbar spine into convexity on the side of contraction and rotate it opposite to the side of contraction.

Signs of weakness: A shortened step and pronounced 'flick' or 'kick' of the lower leg may become apparent when walking. The pelvis, on the side of weakness, will tend to flex anteriorly and rotate internally causing a compensatory posterior flexion and lateral rotation of the opposite pelvis. A potentially harmful compensatory twisting and untwisting of the entire spine develops.

Unilateral weakness: Lumbar scoliosis and a possible anterior flexion of the ilium combined with a functional long leg.

Bilateral weakness: Decreased lordosis of the lumbar spine.

Test

Supine position

The leg is extended at the knee and laterally rotated. At this point it is flexed approximately 40° at the hip and abducted about 30°. As soon as the test position is reached, the patient is told to hold the weight of the leg and then the test is immediately performed as described below.

Stabilization: At the opposite pelvis making sure that it the contact causes no discomfort.

Test contact: The hand that brought the leg to the test position is quickly moved to the distal, medial leg, just above the medial malleolus. The contact should be broad and elicit no pain.

Patient: Presses upwards and slightly towards the midline against the examiner's hand, to bring the leg into flexion and slight adduction. It may be necessary to have one or more 'dry runs' or 'rehearsals' prior to the actual test to make sure the patient understands the correct movement required. Weakness may be already suspected, should the patient display difficulty in holding the leg in the test position. The contact hand may be moved closer to the knee in weaker patients.

Seated position

The hip is flexed to 90° while seated and then abducted to 20°. At this point the femur is laterally rotated so that the foot is moved toward the midline. The patient must hold the lumbar spine in a neutral position to prevent any increase in flexion or lordosis.

Stabilization: Contact to the contralateral shoulder to prevent anterior displacement of the trunk.

Contact: Close to the knee on the distal, slightly medial thigh.

Patient: Pulls the knee diagonally upwards toward the opposite shoulder.

Examiner: Resists by pushing the leg diagonally downwards and somewhat laterally.

Note: If there is functional scoliosis of the lumbar spine, it may be wise to test the various fibres of the muscle. If the scoliosis

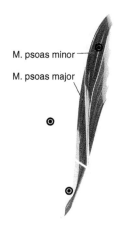

M. psoas minor

M. psoas major

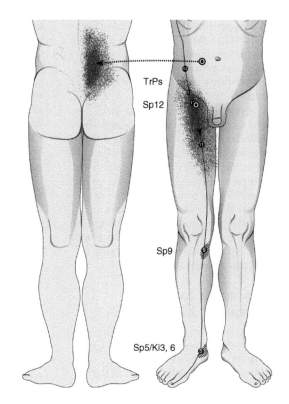

TrPs

Sp12

Sp9

Sp5/Ki3, 6

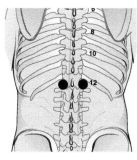

Ki1

Ki7

Referred pain and effective distal points

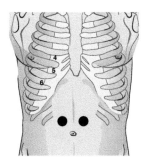

NL posterior

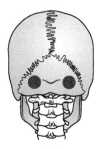

NL anterior

NV

Motor function innervation: Lumbar plexus, L1, L2, L3, L4
Visceroparietal segment (TS line): T11, T12
Rib pump: Intercostal space, costotransverse joint 4, 7 and 12
Organ: Kidneys
Nutrients: Vitamins A and E, water
Meridian: Kidneys
SRS: L1–L5

is in the upper lumbar spine, the leg is abducted to about 20° in order to isolate primarily the superior fibres. When the scoliosis is limited to the lower lumbars, the lower fibres are best isolated by abducting the leg beyond 30°.

Test errors, precautions: Too little lateral rotation of the leg and insufficient stabilization of the pelvis, causing rotation of the pelvis. Less than full extension of the knee by the patient will more often than not cause a false negative test. Any painful contact with the testing hand must be avoided. When muscle weakness is apparent, the adductor muscles should be tested as well. The adductors act as fixators for the hip and when weak will cause a false-positive weakness.

Frequently found associated disorders

A lateral subluxation of the talus has been linked to psoas weakness. An increased pronation of the foot by the testing hand contact, especially in club or flat footedness, may lead to a false weakness of the psoas due to the adverse stimulus from the ankle.

Myofascial syndrome

Stretch test: The patient is placed supine with the buttock on the side to be stretched at the edge of the table. The opposite knee is grasped and drawn up towards the abdomen to stabilize the pelvis posteriorly. The patient is then instructed to keep the knee bent and allow the tested leg to drop over the side of the table.

Shortening of the iliopsoas is indicated when the thigh does not drop below the table surface. If the lower leg does not appear to be almost perpendicular to the floor. This is due to a shortening of the rectus femoris. A shortened tensor fasciae latae may also be the cause.

When trigger points are present, stretch of the iliopsoas will induce referred pain in the area of the SI joint. Stretch can be increased in these cases by placing the leg in full medial rotation and 30° abduction (Travell and Simons 1992).

PIR: From the stretch position and with a sustained inspiration, the patient lifts the knee very slightly. The lower leg remains bent at the knee and must remain hanging loosely downwards throughout the procedure to prevent unwanted, synergistic contraction of the rectus femoris. The relaxation phase the leg is allowed to drop down by its own weight during expiration. The examiner's leg may also push on the patient's lower leg during the relaxation phase to induce more medial rotation of the hip.

When a significant shortening of the rectus femoris is noted, one must relax it first. In difficult cases, the knee and leg may be supported in extension by the examiner. Keeping the leg in extension, the patient is instructed to breathe in and lift the leg. This is followed by the examiner gently lowering the leg as the patient breathes out.

An alternative method for relaxation of the psoas may be made by placing the patient supine and with the examiner palpating the tensed psoas. The patient is asked to attempt, in a relaxed manner, to flex and extend the hips by sliding the heel on the table back and forth on the table. This may be repeated as often as necessary.

Causes for compression: Compression of the iliohypogastric, the ilioinguinal, the lateral femoral cutaneous and the femoral nerves are common. These nerves all exit at the lateral margin of the psoas major or, in the case of the obturator nerve, at the medial margin. The genitofemoral nerve runs through the belly of the muscle and, in some individuals, the iliohypogastric and ilioinguinal nerves as well. Sensory aberrations and pain in the inguinal area, around the scrotum, the labia major and on the anterior thigh are often noted.

Entrapment may also be found in the muscular space of the retroinguinal compartment, where the femoral and genitofemoral nerves exit the pelvis together with the psoas muscle in cases of hypertrophy of the iliopsoas muscle because it is still plump in this area, (Travell and Simons 1992, Lewit 1992).

Frequently found associated disorders

A psoas weakness or a hyporeaction associated with kidney dysfunction is

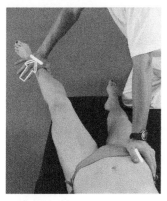

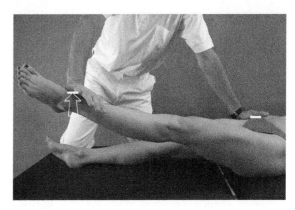

Supine psoas test   Supine psoas test

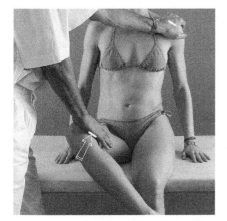

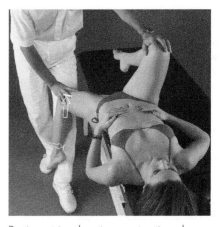

Seated psoas test   Postisometric relaxation, contraction phase

common. In case of metabolic and/or visceral problems of the kidney, the muscle frequently tests weak. Lumbar disorders of any kind may also be attributed to psoas weakness patterns. In cases where lumbar problems are suspected, the test should be performed with some caution. The psoas test alone can lead to an increase in disc symptoms similar to those seen with incorrectly executed 'sit-ups'. The leg is so heavy that the long lever puts additional strain on already weakened and inflamed discs. In these cases, the patient is often unable to obtain or maintain the initial test position due to pain. Bilateral psoas

weakness has been clinically linked to an occipito-atlanto micro-fixation.

Psoas hypertonus is common and most often associated with disorders of the kidney, the cecum on the right and the sigmoid colon on the left. Psoas hypertonus may also provoke unilateral or bilateral inguinal pain.

A hypertonic psoas may eventually lead to a posterior displacement of the ilium, as the muscle runs in front of the axis of the SI joint and stabilizes it anteriorly (Travell and Simons 1992). Talus subluxations, as noted above, are associated with functional psoas weakness.

Anatomy

Origin: Lateral margin of the ischial tuberosity.

Course: From medial to lateral. It is the most inferior placed lateral rotator of the hips.

Insertion: At the intertrochanteric crest.

Action

Lateral rotation in the hip joint and with hip flexion, abduction is noted. When the hips are in neutral position the muscle has a minor adduction and extension function (Frick et al. 1992a).

Test

The following test is the most specific available for the quadratus femoris. No supine test is able to isolate the quadratus femoris from any of the other lateral hip rotators.

Position: The knee is flexed to 90°, the leg adducted to 30° and laterally rotated so that the foot is moved in a medial direction toward the midline of the body.

Stabilization: The lateral aspect of the knee.

Test contact: Medially on the distal part of the patient's lower leg.

Patient: Presses the foot in a medial direction.

Examiner: Resists by pushing the foot laterally.

Test errors, precautions: In prone position too little adduction so that it is not differentiated from the other lateral rotators, especially the piriformis.

Myofascial syndrome

Stretch test: With the patient supine, the thigh is maximally flexed, adducted and medially rotated. Isolating the stretch to the quadratus femoris alone is not possible.

PIR: From the stretch position the patient holds an inspiration and slowly pushes the leg into abduction and lateral rotation. This is followed by the relaxation phase, where the patient breathes out as the examiner gently elongates the muscle by bringing it back to the stretch position.

Frequently found associated disorders

The close relationship of the lateral rotators of the hip means that they have many common and simultaneous lesions. They are typically inhibited singly or in pairs by local origin–insertion problems or by vertebral lesions.

As they are all synergistic they can develop hypertonicity patterns, possibly of the strain-counterstrain type.

Their paired counterparts on the contralateral side can, as a consequence of dysfunction, develop myofascial lesions and shortening as one would see in other antagonist groups.

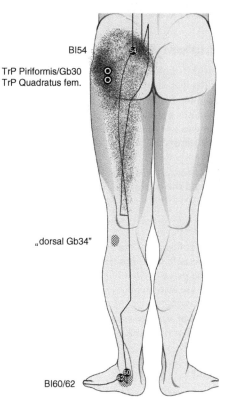

BI54

TrP Piriformis/Gb30
TrP Quadratus fem.

M. piriformis
M. gemellus sup.
M. gemellus inf.
M. obturatorius ext.
M. obturatorius internus
M. quadratus femoris

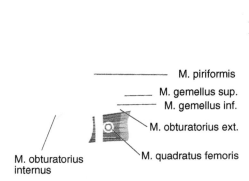

„dorsal Gb34"

BI60/62

Trigger points and effective distal points

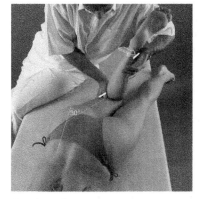

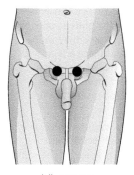

Quadratus femoris test

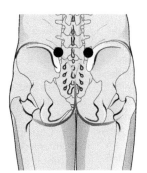

NL anterior

NL posterior

NV

Motor function innervation: Sacral plexus, L5, S1, S2
Visceroparietal segment (TS line): L5
Organ: Gonads
Nutrients: Vitamins B3, E, PUFA, Zn, Se, Mg
Meridian: Pericardium (circulation-sex)
SRS: L5

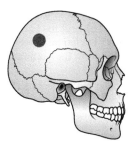

Pe7

Pe9

Anatomy

Origin: Iliolumbar ligament and inner lip of the iliac crest.

Course: Lies in the deepest layer of the posterior muscles of the trunk, almost as if it was a lateral continuation of the intertransverse muscles of the lumbar spine.

Insertion: At the lower margin of the 12th rib and the transverse processes of L1 to L4.

Action

Lateral flexion of the lumbar spine and is the muscle that joins the posterior thorax to the pelvis. When bilaterally contracting they are also auxiliary muscles for forced expiration.

Signs of weakness: Rotation and lateral flexion of the lumbar spine to the opposite side.

Test

Position: The supine patient grasps the table with both hands. The legs are approximated and moved 30–45° towards the side being tested. The patient will now have a bow-like shape or curve with the concavity on the side being tested.

Test contact: The examiner stands opposite the side being tested. With the forearm placed under the distal part of both legs and the hand curled around to grasp the lateral aspect of the leg farthest away from the examiner.

Stabilization: On the side of convexity, closest to the examiner, the free hand is placed on, or about, the area of the greater trochanter. This position allows for stabilization close to the axis of rotation.

Patient: Draws the legs away from the examiner and toward the tested muscle side.

Examiner: Resists both with the testing and stabilizing hands simultaneously.

Test errors, precautions: Lack of stabilization of the patient's trunk so that the body shifts or slides during the test and allowing the patient to lift the legs up from the table surface in order to bring the posterior part of the obliquus abdominis into the test. No pelvic rotation should be allowed.

Myofascial syndrome

Stretch test: The patient sits on the treatment table with the examiner standing behind. On the side opposite to that being stretched, one knee is placed next to the patient's pelvis. With the arm on the tested side lifted over the head, the patient's trunk is laterally bent over the examiner's thigh. This helps to stabilize the pelvis from elevating off the table. Additional stretch may be obtained by adding a flexion component to the trunk.

PIR: From the stretch position the patient is asked to breathe in, and while holding the inspiration, look up with the eyes. This eye position leads to a minimal contraction of the quadratus lumborum. As the patient breathes out and moves the gaze downward, the examiner gently emphasizes the stretch position further using the arm as a lever.

Frequently found associated disorders

Muscle shortening, hypertonicity and trigger points often occur as a consequence of weakness found in the gluteus maximus muscle. Unilateral weakness may induce functional scoliosis and place adverse mechanical stress on the intervertebral discs and the posterior facet joints, as well as provoking compensatory pelvic lesions.

Gluteus maximus weakness will cause an anterior ilium, a high pelvis, and concavity of the lumbar spine on the same side. A compensatory, relative shortening of the quadratus lumborum will be found on the side of gluteus maximus weakness.

When a functional, compensatory lumbar scoliosis is deemed to be caused by an SOT type category I or II pelvic lesion, the applied kinesiology approach will be to treat any weak pelvic stabilizers first, prior any mechanical correction. In this case the

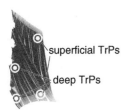

superficial TrPs

deep TrPs

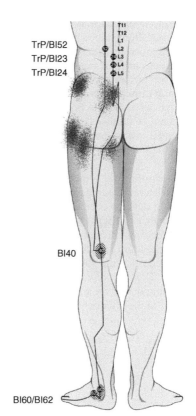

TrP/Bl52
TrP/Bl23
TrP/Bl24

T11
T12
L1
L2
L3
L4
L5

Bl40

Bl60/Bl62

Referred pain and effective distal points

Motor function innervation: Lumbar plexus,
T12 to L3
Visceroparietal segment (TS line): L2
Rib pump: Intercostal space, costotransverse
joint 11
Organ: Large intestine
Nutrients: Vitamins A, C and E
SRS: Thoracic spine, SI joint

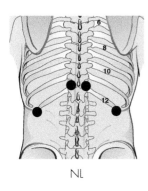

6
8
10
12

NL

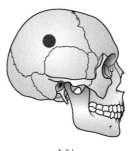

NV

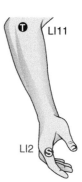

LI11

LI2

functionally weak quadratus lumborum on the posterior ilium side would be treated. Functional muscle weaknesses or hyporeactions are best treated with the aid of the seven factors of the viscerosomatic system and muscle techniques designed to correct the pelvic lesions. Should this protocol not be followed, the hypertonic, contralateral quadratus lumborum will not relax and any trigger points will remain active.

With a chronic unilateral weakness, the contralateral quadratus lumborum will tend to develop compensatory hypertonicity and trigger points.

Myogelosis disturbances in the muscle may pull the ilium anterior on the same side and induce a functional leg length difference. This may be come self-perpetuating due to the mechanisms associated to the high pelvis.

Anatomical leg length differences place undue stress on the SI joint. When instability and/or irritation is present in the SI joint, tender points develop near the insertion of the muscle on the 12th rib.

It might be the case that a permanent solution is only possible after the leg difference has been corrected. After AK compatibility testing, a heel lift may be inserted into the shoe of the short leg side. Functional testing is critically important. Trying to equalize the leg length when there is a fixed, structural scoliosis may lead to further deterioration. The midline axis of the body could even deviate further from the midline rather than returning to a symmetrical balance. According to Travell and Simons (1983), attempting to straighten the spine in this way may actually impart increased structural stress into the vertebral column.

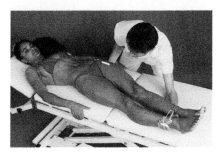

Quadratus lumborum test

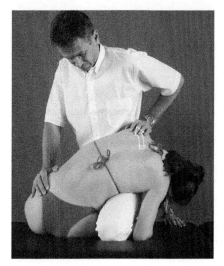

PIR of quadratus lumborum: contraction phase, inspiration

Anatomy

Origin: M. rectus femoris: Anterior inferior spina iliaca.

M. vastus intermedius: Below the intertrochanteric line on the anterior surface of the femur.

M. vastus lateralis: Base of the greater trochanter and lateral part of the linea aspera.

M. vastus medialis: Distal part of the intertrochanteric line and medial part of the linea aspera.

Course: All muscles from superior to inferior and they form the anterior profile of the thigh. The vastus intermedius lies deep to, and is completely covered by, the rectus femoris.

Insertion: All divisions converge into a common tendon that inserts over the patella and the patellar ligament, ending at the tibial tuberosity.

Action

Flexes the hip and extends the knee joint. After the ball of the foot has pushed off from the ground and the leg is still in extension, the rectus femoris is the main agonist (initiator) of the forward movement of the femur. The pull from the psoas changes at this angle due to being stretched over the pubic bone and will not have a strong pulling effect.

Together with the vastus medialis, intermedius and lateralis it extends the knee. The vastus medialis, especially the more distal vastus medialis obliquus portion, stabilizes the patella medially and the vastus lateralis stabilizes the patella laterally.

Signs of weakness: A low pelvis on the side of the weakness is due to posterior rotation of the ilium. A shortened step might be noted, but more often than not the pelvis and leg will swing together. No smooth transition of the leg is forthcoming as it seems fixed on the pelvis. Difficulty is also apparent in climbing and descending stairs, in standing up from a sitting position or sitting down from a standing position. The body must lean forward in order to make these movements and the arms are classically used for support.

Test

Rectus femoris in the seated position
This evaluates the flexion capacity at the hip. While both the rectus femoris and the psoas have strong actions in this position, the action of the rectus femoris has a clearly different vector than that of the psoas which flexes, adducts and externally rotates the hip when in 90° of flexion. Careful attention to the degree of hip flexion is important.

Position: Lift the thigh no more than about a hand's width from the treatment table.

Stabilization: In some cases, extra care should be taken in stabilization of the trunk by holding the ipsilateral shoulder to prevent any forward displacement of the trunk during the test.

Test contact: On the top of the distal thigh, close to the knee.

Patient: Draws the knee up towards the shoulder on the same side.

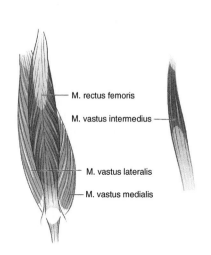

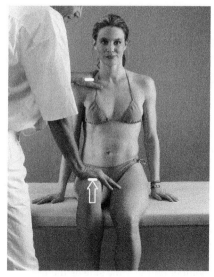

Seated rectus femoris test

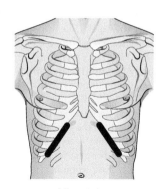

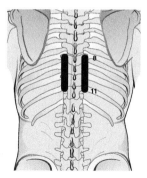

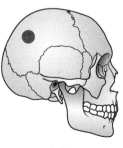

NL anterior   NL posterior   NV

Motor function innervation: Femoral nerve, L2, L3, L4
Visceroparietal segment (TS line): T10
Rib pump: Intercostal space, costotransverse joint 1, 4, 6, 7, 8
Organ: Small intestine
Nutrients: Ca, vitamin-B-complex, vitamin D, probiotics, coenzyme Q10
Meridian: Small intestine
SRS:
Rectus femoris: L1
Vastus lateralis and medialis: L2
Vastus intermedius: L3

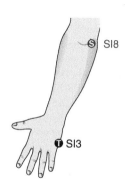

Classic test: rectus femoris test supine (effect on hip joint)

Position: The knee is flexed to 90° and the hip is flexed preferably, especially in strong patients, to about 70°, but less than 90°.

Test contact: On the distal femur, proximal to the knee.

Stabilization: Usually this is not critical as the trunk is relatively stabilized in this position. On examination tables having a slick surface, sliding of the body may occur as a consequence of the strong resisting forces made by the examiner. It may be necessary to stabilize the patient with the non-testing hand over the contralateral leg or by having the patient grasp the table with one or both hands.

Patient: Draws the knee towards the shoulder on the same side as the test.

Examiner: Resists in a direction that will bring the knee down towards the other knee, following a vector along the arc of movement of the knee as the femur descends towards the table.

Alternative, supine rectus femoris test

Position: The supine patient flexes the hip no more than 10° and the knee is held slightly off full extension. The very strong psoas will enter the test when flexion is greater than 15°. A full or 'locked in' extension of the knee will activate the obliquus portion of the medialis as well as the other vasti. Any reactive muscle patterns or knee joint dysfunction may reflexively weaken the muscle; thus keeping the knee slightly off full extension is important.

Stabilization: If necessary, the pelvis on the other side, although it is best to use both hands for accurate testing.

Test contact: To the distal leg with one hand and with the other hand, just above the slightly bent knee.

Patient: Pushes the leg up while keeping the knee slightly off full extension.

Examiner: Resists elevation of the leg. Care should be taken because the lever is

very long and it is very easy to overpower the limb. Note, too, that more resistance is imparted at the contact just above the knee and less pressure distally.

Should the above test be made with the knee in full extension and the vastus medialis muscle contracted, a general test of knee extension stability will be made. Therefore, should the test be normal with the knee slightly flexed, but weak with the knee in full extension, it is indicative of some dysfunction in full knee extension. A weakness reaction may be due to knee joint receptor problems, reactive muscle interaction between the muscles acting on the joint, or any other stabilization problem. A more detailed discussion of this testing procedure can be found below.

It is best that the test be confirmed by comparing it with the basic test for the vastus group.

Seated group test: vastus lateralis, intermedius, medialis and rectus femoris (effect on knee joint)

Position: The knee flexed to about 45° over the edge of the table. In very strong patients, the leg may be flexed even more. Allowing too much extension will almost always negate any weakness finding due the inherent strength of the muscles. Pain may be noted at the back of the knee during testing. The examiner's free hand may be placed on the table surface with the hollow of the leg resting upon it to provide a cushion.

Test contact: On the distal, anterior aspect of the lower leg.

Stabilization: On the anterior aspect of the ipsilateral shoulder.

Patient: Pulls the foot up against the resistance from the examiner.

Supine group test: vastus lateralis, intermedius, medialis and rectus femoris (effect on knee joint)

This test is not recommended when the patient is extremely strong and/or the

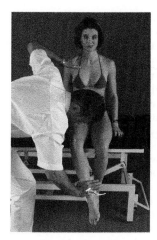
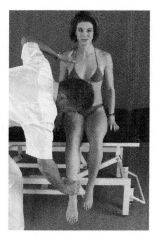
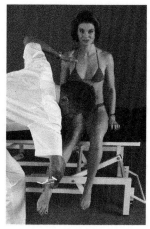

Vastus lateralis test
Observe the test vector: The
examiner holds into knee
flexion and external rotation of
the thigh

Quadriceps femoris test

Vastus medialis test
Observe the test vector: The
examiner holds into knee
flexion and further internal
rotation of the thigh

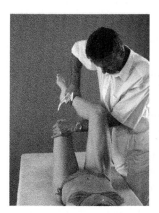
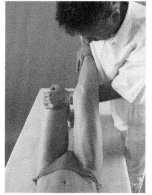
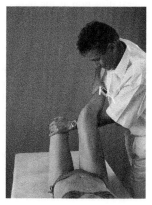

Vastus lateralis test
Observe the test vector: The
examiner holds into knee
flexion and external rotation of
the thigh

Quadriceps femoris test

Vastus medialis test
Observe the test vector: The
examiner holds into knee
flexion and internal rotation of
the thigh

forearm of the examiner is not sufficiently robust to resist the resistance pressures during the test.

Position: Flex the hip of the non-tested leg to about 45° and place the foot firmly on the table surface. The examiner firmly grasps the knee with one hand so that the forearm forms a sort of bridge. The hollow of the knee of the tested leg is placed on the forearm with the knee flexed about a 45° angle.

Patient: Pushes the foot up against the resisting hand of the examiner.

Vastus medialis test (seated or supine)

From any of the above starting positions, the hip is medially rotated about 15° so that the foot moves laterally, away from the midline. The test contact changes on the distal leg and is placed over the anterior aspect of the medial malleolus. The examiner resists in a direction to further flex the knee and in a slightly lateral direction as the patient pushes the lower leg up to extend the knee.

Vastus lateralis test

The hips are laterally rotated 15° (the foot is moved medially). Contact is made on the anterior aspect of the lateral malleolus. The examiner resists so as to further flex the knee and in a slightly medial direction as the patient pushes the lower leg up to extend the knee

Test errors, precautions: When testing the rectus femoris as a hip flexor with the patient in supine position, excess pressure on the common tendon at the superior margin of the patella may cause pain and stimulate tendon receptors, both of which can cause concomitant weakening of the muscle. This may also occur when using a testing vector, which does not follow the arc of movement described by the knee during hip flexion.

Vastus medialis pars obliqua (VMO)

Especially when dealing with cases of patellofemoral syndrome, normal functioning of the distal (oblique) part of the vastus medialis (VMO) is crucial. Medial stabilization of the patella when the knee is fully extended is severely reduced when the VMO is weakened or inhibited.

The VMO is almost impossible to test directly due to the strong synergism of the rectus and vasti. An indirect, modified testing procedure may be beneficial.

The procedure uses the rectus femoris response to full knee extension. The VMO is of paramount importance for medial knee stability during full extension. Weakness or hypertonus of the VMO will stimulate knee joint nociceptors and subsequently weaken the rectus muscle. It must be noted here that the procedure evaluates knee extension stability, to which the VMO contributes, but it is not a single entity for stability. The full knee extension test will evaluate the combined activity of the VMO, and the other quadriceps divisions as well. Even though the vasti extend the knee, they have no direct effect on the hip. Reactive patterns between the divisions, however, may cause rectus femoris weakness. The cause of the inhibition can be found by TL over the knee joint and the muscles acting on it. An area, whose TL eliminates the weakness may be considered as responsible for the positive test.

Step one: Evaluation of normal rectus femoris function. Raise the almost fully extended leg about 10–15° above the surface of the table. Keep the knee off full extension. If found strong (normo-reactive), proceed to step two. If weak, the muscle must be evaluated and treated before progressing to step two.

Step two: The above test is repeated, yet this time with maximum extension of the knee. For this test, contact is made to the distal leg with the one hand and a light contact with the other hand just above the knee. This allows one to also palpate the contraction of the VMO. About 60–70% of the resistance pressure is made with the hand pressing above the knee and the remaining 30–40% is made by the distal hand. This will keep the examiner from overpowering the muscle.

It is critical that the patient maintain full extension of the knee during the test. Permitting even 1–2° of flexion will often be enough to negate any weakness. Should the patient have a problem that is

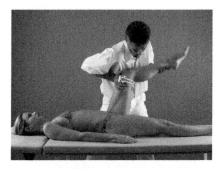

Supine rectus femoris test. Note: The rectus femoris is very strong. Considerable resistance using body weight may be required

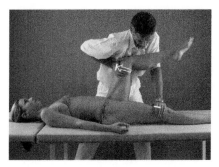

Correct resistance vectors will reduce sliding of the body. Sliding may be restricted by stabilizing the contralateral leg with the other hand

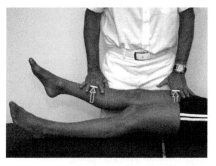

Rectus femoris test with extensor challenge on the knee joint

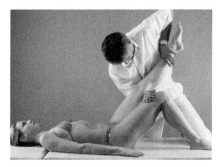

Quadriceps test with patellar compression challenge

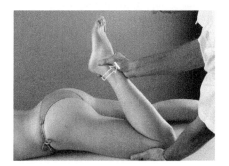

Stretch test and contraction phase of the PIR for the rectus femoris

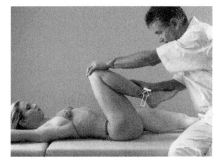

PIR of the vastus group: contraction phase

evidenced in full extension, the ability to maintain full extension is reduced or almost lost. Therefore, patients will tend to very slightly flex the knee, unconsciously sensing that it will improve resistance strength. The examiner must constantly monitor the VMO for contraction during the testing procedure by palpating the muscle with the stabilizing hand.

Myofascial syndrome

Stretch test: With the patient in the prone position the rectus femoris is selectively isolated when the knee is maximally flexed. In the absence of knee joint restriction, and if the tone and length of the rectus femoris are normal, the heel should reach the patient's buttock with ease.

Vastus group: With the patient in the supine position and the hip flexed to 90°, the leg is fully flexed at the knee. The rectus femoris is effectively removed from the test as it will elongate further at the knee due to hip flexion. As with the above test, the patient's heel should be able to touch the buttock with ease.

During the stretch test trigger points may be activated with classic referred pain symptoms. When trigger points are present, the quadriceps group will be found to be weak during normal testing or, following stretch. Weakness can also be concluded in those individuals whereby the knee suddenly bends or gives way without provocation when standing or walking. Trigger points in the vastus medialis and the vastus lateralis will cause asymmetrical tracking of the patella along the femoropatellar articular surface.

PIR: During the relaxation phase of PIR where the patient is in the supine position and the hip in extension, the psoas cannot be isolated from the rectus femoris. As described above, the rectus femoris may be selectively elongated when the patient is prone. Without inducing pain, the heel is brought towards the buttock as far as possible and held there by the examiner. During a sustained inspiration, the patient lightly presses the lower leg into extension against the examiner's gentle resistance. As the patient breathes out, the examiner brings the leg back to the start position and can enhance the stretch by taking the leg slightly beyond the initial tissue resistance point. Patients can also perform this exercise alone.

The vastus group is treated in the supine position with the hip flexed to 90° and the knee maximally flexed. The patient holds the distal aspect of the leg against the buttock or as close as is possible to it. Again under a sustained inspiration, the patient releases the leg and extends the knee by pushing the foot lightly and gradually into the hands of the examiner. During the relaxation phase, the patient slowly exhales while gently returning the knee to the stretch position.

Frequently found associated disorders

Pelvic instability, knee instability, gait disorders, difficulty standing up from a seated position and climbing stairs. Retropatellar arthrosis and inhibition of the vastus group are frequently associated because of faulty patellar tracking.

Compression weakness: Inguinal ligament iliopsoas syndrome, lumbar disc lesions at L2/3 involving the L3 root and weakening both the rectus femoris and the psoas. This will be noted most readily in hip flexion. Note that patellar tendon reflex inhibition is only produced by L4 (Patten 1998).

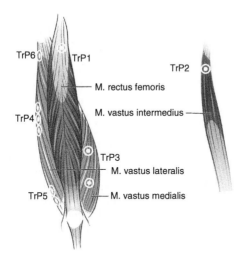

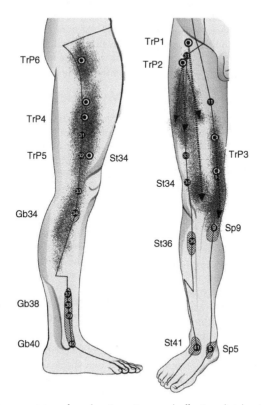

Trigger points, referred pain pattern and effective distal points

Anatomy

Origin: Rhomboideus minor: Nuchal ligament, spinous processes of the vertebrae C7 and T1.

Rhomboideus major: From the spinous processes of T2–5 and the supraspinous ligament.

Course: Laterally and slightly inferior to the medial margin of the scapula.

Insertion: Rhomboideus minor: On the medial margin of the scapula at the level of the scapular spinous process.

Rhomboideus major: On the medial margin of the scapula caudal to the scapular spinous process.

Action

Both muscles rotate, retract and adduct the scapula. They also aid in elevating the medial border of the scapula and in fixating the medial border of the scapula to the spine and thorax. The movement of the scapula is medial causing the glenoid cavity to rotate inferiorly.

Signs of weakness: Protraction of the shoulder with the space between the spinous process of the spine and the medial border of the scapula enlarged. During abduction of the arm, a lack of stabilization of the scapula is noted. When lifting or lowering the arm, a slight back and forth swinging movement of the arm may be noted between 40 and 120° of abduction.

Test

Position: With the forearm in supination, the elbow is flexed to at least 90°, placed close to the trunk slightly behind the midline of the thorax. This aids in keeping the shoulder retracted as the patient is instructed to bring the medial margin of the scapula to the vertebral column, i.e. draws the shoulder back and up.

Test contact: The palm of the testing hand contacts the elbow and the fingers are curled around to contact its medial aspect.

Note: Contact should be made with the most anterior hand with respect to the patient as this will automatically create a slightly anterior resistance vector.

Stabilization: The free hand stabilizes the shoulder by contacting the humeral head superiorly and laterally.

Patient: Holds the elbow against the trunk and draws the shoulders back in the direction of the vertebral column.

Examiner: Pulls the elbow away from the body in a lateral and somewhat anterior and superior direction.

Test errors, precautions: Lack of retraction and elevation of the scapula at the start of the test. Allowing the patient to pull the elbow anteriorly, bring the shoulder flexors into the test and should the examiner not follow the resistance vector. This test is very similar to that of the levator scapula. Therefore, it is only the scapular movement pattern that will be indicative of the muscle causing the weakness. For example, descent of the superior, medial angle of the scapula without enlarging the vertebral-medial scapular border space, is indicative of levator scapular weakness. Descent of the medial angle and enlargement of the space indicates rhomboid weakness.

Myofascial syndrome

Stretch test: The upper arm and the shoulder are brought as far as possible to the anterior of the body and the shoulder is depressed maximally. The medial scapular border should be moved away from the vertebral column.

PIR: From the stretch position, the patient is asked to pull the shoulder back and draw it up during a prolonged inspiration. During expiration the examiner gently returns the limb and shoulder to the stretch position and then a bit farther.

Frequently found associated disorders

Strain-counterstrain and reactive muscle lesions following direct injuries or due to a sudden shock absorption by the arm and shoulder during falls is common, as well as a spondylogenic reflex pattern from the lower cervicals reflecting to the shoulder.

Compression weaknesses: C4 root syndrome (intervertebral foramen C3/C5) and scalenus syndrome.

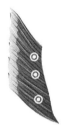

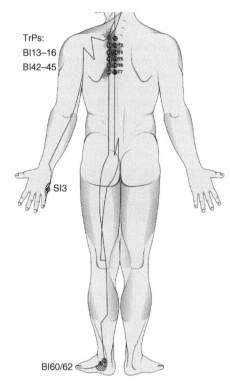

TrPs:
Bl13–16
Bl42–45

SI3

C4
C5
C6
C7
Th1
Th2

Bl60/62

Trigger points and effective distal points

Spondylogenic reflex zones

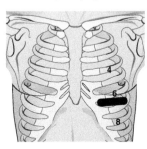

NL anterior

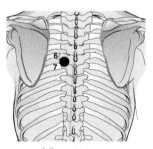

NL posterior

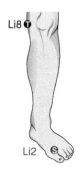

Li8

Li2

Motor function innervation:
Dorsal scapular nerve, C4, C5
Organ: Liver
Meridian: Liver
Nutrients: Vitamin A, lipotropic
factors such as choline, inositol,
l-methionine, glutathione and
sulphur donors such as cysteine
(detoxification metabolism)
SRS: C4–T2

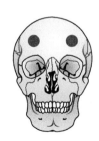

Test of the rhomboids

NV

The muscles associated with the sacrospinal system are the longissimus and the iliocostalis, while the paraspinous muscles belong to the transversospinal system: M. multifidus and mm. rotatores longi and brevis.

The medial m. longissimus consists of the longissimus lumborum, longissimus thoracis, longissimus capitis and longissimus cervicis.

The m. iliocostalis represents the lateral part of the erector spinae (sacrospinalis) and can be divided into the iliocostalis lumborum, iliocostalis thoracis and iliocostalis cervicis.

M. iliocostalis cervicis

Anatomy

Origin: On the medial aspect of the costal angles of the 3rd to 7th ribs.

Course: Runs lateral to the longissimus cervicis and capitis, medial to the scalenus posterior and medius, and medial to the levator scapulae.

Insertion: Together with the longissimus cervicis on the posterior tubercle of the transverse processes 3rd to 6th cervical vertebrae.

M. iliocostalis thoracis

Anatomy

Origin: On the medial costal angle of the 7th to 12th ribs.

Course: Lateral to the longissimus cervicis and capitis.

Insertion: On the lateral aspect and upper edge of the costal angle of the 1st to 7th ribs and sometimes into the posterior part of the transverse process of C7.

M. iliocostalis lumborum

Anatomy

Origin: Together with the longissimus at the sacrum and on the ventrolateral surface of the iliac tuberosity.

Course: Runs lateral to the longissimus thoracis.

Insertion: On the inferior edges of the angles of the 4th to 12th ribs.

M. iliocostalis (all divisions)

Action

Bilateral contraction extends the vertebral column.

One-sided contraction laterally flexes the vertebral column to the same side.

Test

The possibility of isolating of one of the above muscles from the rest of the back extensors is extremely doubtful at best.

Beardall (1980), however, does describe a test for the iliocostalis lumborum. The patient is placed supine with the upper body laterally flexed to about 10° to the tested side. The leg on the side of trunk flexion is fully medially rotated.

With the patient in a position similar to that for the oblique and transverse abdominals, the examiner stands or sits opposite the side to be tested. One hand contacts and stabilizes the lateral border of the pelvis closest to the examiner. The testing arm slides underneath both legs, as distal as is possible, until the fingers can curl upward and around to contact the medially rotated leg. When positioning is achieved, the patient is instructed to pull both legs away from the examiner while the examiner exerts opposite resistance.

Myofascial syndrome

Stretch test (back extensors as a group): The patient stands with the legs spread apart to about shoulder width and is asked to laterally bend the trunk first to one side, then the other. The sides are compared visually for any deviations in symmetrical movement.

PIR: Starting with the feet apart as above, the patient stands with the upper body bent forward and the spine arched as much as is comfortably possible. This is very similar to the touching the finger to ground evaluation for hamstring contraction.

While in this stretch position, a deep inspiration taken and held for 10 seconds. Inspiration causes the back extensors to tense. The body is kept in the same position for the relaxation phase while the patient exhales slowly. Elongation of the muscles is made by body weight alone.

If desired, in order to increase the therapeutic effect during the relaxation phase, the patient may slightly flex the body to one side or the other. This will tend to favour elongation of the extensors on the opposite side.

Or, as an alternative to performing PIR in the forward flexed position, one may execute PIR from the lateral inclination 'stretch' position as described in the 'stretching' section above. This will isolate the muscles on one side. While sustaining an inspiration, the patient slowly returns to an upright position. The relaxation phase is made with the patient breathing out while the trunk is slowly returned to the starting position.

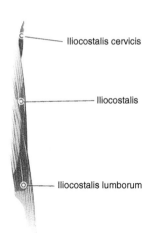

- Iliocostalis cervicis
- Iliocostalis
- Iliocostalis lumborum

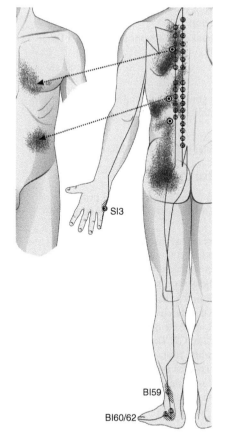

SI3

BI59

BI60/62

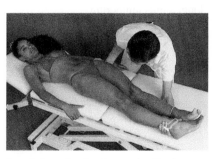

Beardall test for the iliocostalis. The leg on the side of the tested muscle must be medially rotated

Trigger points and effective distal points of the iliocostalis muscle. Pain is referred into the segment in a more kaudal and ventral direction

M. longissimus capitis

Anatomy

Origin: From the transverse processes C5 to C7 (to T1 to T3).

Course: In a superior direction from the origin, it is bordered medially by the longissimus cervicis and laterally by the semispinalis capitis.

Insertion: In an area of about 1.5 cm at the posterior margin of the mastoid process as far as its tip and deep to both the splenius capitis and sternocleidomastoid muscles.

Action

One-sided contraction: Inclination and rotation of the head towards the side of contraction.

Bilateral contraction: Extension of the head.

Test

Only a general test of all the neck extensors is possible.

M. longissimus cervicis

Anatomy

Origin: From the transverse processes of T1 to T6 and in some cases as far down as T8.

Course: From the origin, the lower half lies medial to the longissimus thoracis and ascends to the cervical insertions lateral to the longissimus capitis.

Insertion: At the posterior surface and root of the transverse processes of C2 to C5 and, in some cases, all the cervicals from C1 to C7. The insertions are, in all practicality, found together with those of the iliocostalis cervicis, splenius cervicis, levator scapulae, scalenus posterior and longissimus capitis.

Action

One-sided contraction: Inclination of the cervical spine towards the side of contraction.

Bilateral contraction: Extension of the cervical spine.

Test

Only a general test of the all the neck extensors is possible.

M. longissimus thoracis

Anatomy

Origin: With the longissimus lumborum and the iliocostalis lumborum, it has a common origin on the dorsum, medial and lateral crests of the sacrum and the spinal processes of the lumbar spine.

Course: It is sandwiched between the spinalis muscle laterally and the iliocostalis medially.

Insertion: The medial insertions are on the transverse processes of the thoracic spine, whereas the lateral insertions are on the surface found between the tubercle and the costal angle.

Action

One-sided contraction: Inclination of the vertebral column to the side of contraction.

Bilateral contraction: Extension of the vertebral column.

Test

See longissimus lumborum.

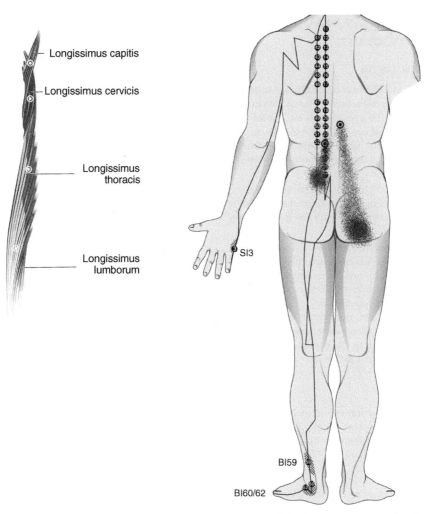

Longissimus capitis

Longissimus cervicis

Longissimus
thoracis

Longissimus
lumborum

SI3

BI59

BI60/62

Trigger points of the longissimus, pain referral
and effective distal points

M. longissimus lumborum

Anatomy

Origin: The muscle originates superficially on the aponeurosis of the sacrospinal system. The aponeurosis has broad bony origins that are derived from the superior and anterior aspects of the iliac tuberosity, the sacrum and the spinous processes of the lumbar spine.

Course: Lying deep to the iliocostalis and the longissimus thoracis muscles, it is closely associated with the interosseous SI ligament.

Insertion: The muscle has a double insertion with two slips each to the mammillary and accessory processes of the lumbar vertebrae. Combined, the insertions form a ligamentous bridge under which run the dorsal rami of the spinal nerves. The lateral fibres arise more deeply and exit to insert at the dorsal surface of the lumbar spinal processes.

Action

One-sided contraction: inclination of the vertebral column. Bilateral contraction: extension of the vertebral column.

Test

Any attempt to isolate the muscle is impossible due to the complex synergistic relationship with other muscles. Nevertheless, the longissimus lumborum may be tested with the patient placed in a supine position with approximately 20° of lateral inclination of the thorax compared to the legs and extended lumbar spine. This corresponds to Goodheart's (in Walther 2000) quadratus lumborum test. Palpation of the muscle together with TL and the use of a SIM appears a more sensible choice.

Myofascial syndrome

Stretch test: The patient is seated with the knees bent so that the hamstring muscles are shortened. The patient is then instructed to bend forward at the waist to check for symmetry and adverse tension. Assessment by having the standing patient perform a lateral inclination may give a more complete picture. The two sides are subsequently compared for any restrictions in movement symmetry.

PIR: The patient stands with the legs spread to about shoulder width and upper body is bent forward as if to try to touch the fingers to the toes. The patient is asked to take a deep inspiration and hold it for about 10 seconds. The act of breathing in will also tense the back extensors. This is followed by a slow expiration that will lead to muscle relaxation. Body weight alone is enough for muscle extension and stretch.

If deemed necessary, a slight rotation to one side or the other will tend to increase the stretch of the extensors on the contralateral side.

Alternatively, one may start from the lateral inclination position as described above. Likewise, deep inspiration will tense the stretched muscles, straightening the spine and expiration relaxes the muscles to return the trunk to the start position.

Cause of compression

Compression can occur in the area of the tendon bridge where the dorsal rami of the spinal nerves can be irritated, leading to hyperaesthesia, dysaesthesia or hypoaesthesia of the skin (Travell and Simons 1992).

Frequently found associated disorders

If an anatomical or functional leg length difference is noted and an adaptative scoliosis present, the back extensor muscles may become overexerted due to postural strains. Correspondingly, a myofascial pain syndrome might develop. A fixed, ideopathic scoliosis is always associated with an imbalance of the back extensors.

Table 1 Spondylogenic reflex syndrome

Tensioned myotones		Lesion segment	Tensioned myotones		Lesion segment
Origin	Insertion		Origin	Insertion	
M. longissimus capitis			M. longissimus thoracis I		
C3	Mastoid process	C7	L3	T5	L1
C4	Mastoid process	T1	L4	T6	L2
C5	Mastoid process	T2	L5	T7	L3
C6	Mastoid process	T3	Sacrum	T8	L4
C7	Mastoid process	T4	Sacrum	T9	L5
T1	Mastoid process	T5	M. longissimus thoracis II		
T2	Mastoid process	T6	Sacrum	T5	T9
T3	Mastoid process	T7	Sacrum	T6	T10
T4	Mastoid process	T8	Sacrum	T7	T11
T5	Mastoid process	T9	Sacrum	T8	T12
M. longissimus cervicis			M. longissimus thoracis III		
T2	C2	C7	Ilium	T8	L1
T3	C2	T1	Ilium	T9	L2
T4	C3	T2	Ilium	T10	L3
T4	C4	T3	Ilium	T11	L4
T5	C5	T4	Ilium	T12	L5
T6	C6	T5	M. longissimus lumborum		
M. longissimus thoracis V			Sacrum, ilium	L1–L3	SI joint
L1	T1	T5	Sacrum, ilium	L1–L5	C7–T4
L2	T2	T6			
L3	T3	T7			
L4	T4	T8			

Spondylogenic reflexes for the longissimus muscle. The origin and insertion of the 'tensioned myotones' are linked to a vertebral segment concluded to be in 'lesion'.

Anatomy

These muscles comprise the deep layer or 'autochthonous' muscles of the back. Also called intrinsic muscles of the spine, they have their origin and insertion on the osseous structures of the spine and ribs.

Origin: Multifidus sacralis: Dorsum of the sacrum, medial surface of the posterior superior iliac spine and posterior part of the SI ligament.

Multifidus lumbalis: Mammillary processes of the lumbar vertebrae.

Multifidus thoracalis: Transverse processes of the thoracic vertebrae and the articular processes of C4–C7.

Course: Obliquely upward and medial. The mass of the muscle fills the groove between the transverse and spinous processes.

Insertion: As a deep fibre bundle two vertebral levels above the origin and with the superficial fibre bundle 3–5 vertebral levels above. All fibres insert on the spinous processes of the relevant vertebrae.

Action

The multifidi help to stiffen the spine and protect the posterior joints from early degeneration.

Bilateral contraction extends the vertebral column.

Unilateral contraction rotates the vertebral column to the opposite side.

Test

Kendall never described a specific test for these muscles. Beardall (1980), however, developed a test for the multifidus lumborum that is very similar to the iliocostalis lumborum test, its only difference lies in the rotation component of the femur. For the iliocostalis femur leg rotation is medial and for the multifidus lumborum it is lateral. The supine patient laterally bends the upper body about 10° to the side being evaluated. The femur is laterally rotated on the tested side.

As with the quadratus lumborum, the examiner stands or sits opposite the side being examined and stabilizes the lateral pelvis with one hand. The other hand and arm pass distally, under both legs, allowing the fingers to curl up, grasping the laterally rotated leg. Alternatively, the examiner may grasp the legs from above, in a similar fashion.

The patient is instructed to draw both legs away from the examiner and towards the side of the test.

Examiner: Resists by pulling the legs out of the lateral flexion position.

Test errors, precautions: The test parameters must be strictly followed. The test is dependent upon the normal functioning of many synergistic muscles, especially the quadratus lumborum, transverse and oblique abdominals. It might be wise to consider testing the synergistic muscles prior to making any definitive conclusion as to which muscle is weakened.

Myofascial syndrome

Stretch test: No isolated stretching possible.

PIR: See sacrospinal system as a group.

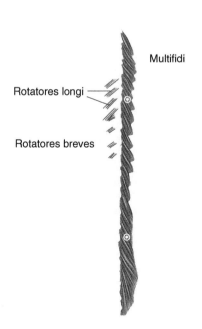

Multifidi

Rotatores longi

Rotatores breves

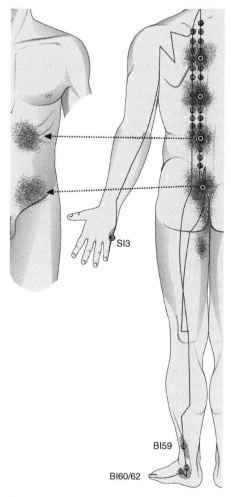

SI3

BI59

BI60/62

Trigger points, referred pain pattern and effective distal points

Motor function innervation: Dorsal rami of the spinal nerves

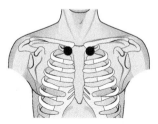

NL anterior: for all autocthonous muscles including the multifidi

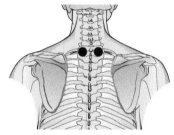

NL posterior: for all autochtonous muscles, including the multifidi

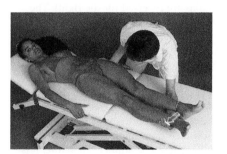

Beardall test for the multifidus lumborum. Note lateral rotation of the leg on the tested side

Anatomy

Origin: On the superior anterior iliac spine.

Course: In a spiralling track crossing from the insertion, down the anterior, then medial thigh, passing behind the medial condyle of the femur to its insertion just below the knee.

Insertion: On the anteromedial surface of the tibia, medial to the tibial tuberosity in the pes anserinus. It is the most anteriorly situated tendon of the pes anserinus whose fibres radiate into the deep fascia of the leg and partly into the patellar ligament.

Action

Abducts, flexes and laterally rotates the femur. It also flexes and medially rotates the tibia, thus allowing for the cross-legged sitting position commonly known as the 'tailor's seat'. The first part of the muscle's name 'sartor' is Latin for tailor.

Signs of weakness: Posterior displacement of the ilium, pain and discomfort over the distal third of the muscle. Lack of medial stabilization of the knee with a possible 'knock kneed' appearance (genu valgum).

Test

Position: Same initial position as for the Faber and Patrick tests. The knee is flexed to approximately 90°, the thigh abducted and flexed so that the heel may be placed at the level of or slightly below the opposite knee.

Test contact: For the left leg (hand positions are reversed for the right). The right hand is placed on the lateral aspect of the knee and the left hand grips the lower leg (close to the medial malleolus of the ankle) from above curling the fingers around and under to get a better purchase on the leg.

Patient: Presses the knee out and down and draws the heel towards the buttocks. The coupled movement is complicated for both patient and examiner. Therefore, it is probably wise to have at least one 'dry run or rehearsal' before the actual test.

In order to correctly perform the test, equal resistance pressure should be made simultaneously by the examiner on the knee and lower leg. Medial pressure should be placed on the knee while the foot and leg are drawn downwards. Especially with strong patients, the test is best made with the examiner's arms locked and with the elbows close to the trunk. Medial torque is made with the examiner's upper body and limb elevation by the strong leg muscles.

Test errors, precautions: The power for the test must be equal and simultaneous from both hands. If too little force is generated by the resisting hand on the knee, in the direction of adduction and medial rotation of the femur, the inferior pull made on the foot will predominantly test the medial hamstrings and not the sartorius. Care should be taken to prevent any contact on the ankle that would provoke pain during the test. This is especially true when a heavy grip is taken over the Achilles tendon.

Myofascial syndrome

Stretch test: The patient lies supine with the buttocks at the edge of the treatment table. The free, non-treated leg is flexed to the chest and held there by the patient to aid in stabilizing the pelvis and the lumbar spine. The leg to be tested is placed in adduction and medial rotation and then extended below the table surface as far as it will naturally go.

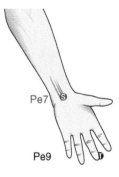

Pe7

Pe9

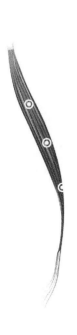

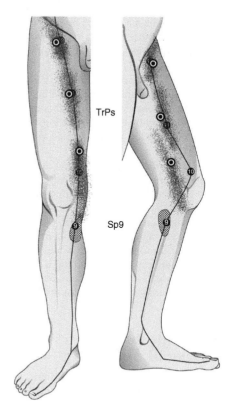

Effective distal point: Sp9

Motor function innervation: Femoral nerve, L2, L3
Visceroparietal segment (TS line): T9
Rib pump zone: Intercostals space, costotransverse joint 9
Organ: Adrenal glands
Nutrients: Adrenal gland extract, tyrosine, vitamins B3, B5, B6, B12, folic acid, vitamin C, manganese, ginseng
Meridian: Pericardium (circulation-sex)
SRS: L3

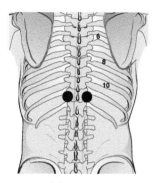

NL posterior

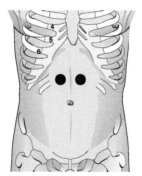

NL anterior

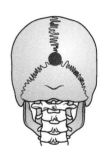

NV

Stretch may be made in the prone position but is more difficult to perform.

PIR: From the stretch position and with a sustained inspiration, the patient is instructed to slowly contract the muscle by flexing, abducting and laterally rotating the leg. As the patient gradually breathes out, the examiner gently elongates the muscle by returning the leg to the original stretch position.

Cause for compression: In some cases, the lateral femoral cutaneous nerve penetrates the sartorius after exiting from the abdomen at a point just below the inguinal ligament. At either point, whether during its passage below the inguinal ligament or through the sartorius muscle, an entrapment can occur resulting in the classic complaint known as lateral femoral cutaneous meralgia paraesthetica (numb or painful thigh).

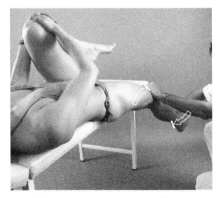

PIR of the sartorius: contraction phase

Frequently found associated disorders

Adrenal gland dysfunction, exhaustion syndrome (burnout), posterior displacement of the ilium causing a consequent SI joint lesion, lack of medial knee stability and medial knee pain.

Compression weakness: L3 root syndrome from the L3/L4 intervertebral foramen, inguinal ligament/iliopsoas syndrome.

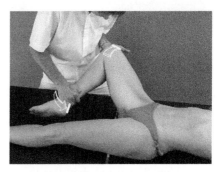

Sartorius test using examiner body torque, legs and arm 'locked'

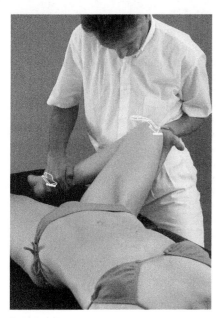

Sartorius test

Anatomy

Origin: From the lateral and superior surfaces of the upper nine ribs.

Insertion: Anterior surface of the scapula near the medial margin.

Action

Stabilizes the scapula while the humerus is elevated into flexion and abduction to a point approximately 90° from the trunk.

As the humerus moves past the 90° point, the serratus abducts and rotates the scapula so that the inferior angle moves laterally and the glenoid cavity rotates superiorly. When the scapulae are fixed, an anterior to posterior movement of the thorax occurs. The muscle stabilizes the scapula on the chest when an anterior to posterior stress is exerted on the arms and out through the shoulder. Classic examples of this would be in performing push-ups or from traumatic insult imparted while gripping the steering wheel during a front-end collision.

Signs of weakness: Posterior pressure on the extended arm and exerted through the shoulders leads to a classic 'winging of the scapula', where the scapula is seen to elevate away from the thorax. In cases of severe weakness the 'winging' is also noted during normal flexion and abduction of the arm. An unnatural 'swinging' movement of the scapula may occur at about 40° of humeral abduction and can be particularly pronounced when lifting and lowering the arm.

Test

Position: With the elbow in extension the humerus is flexed by elevating the arm to a point of about 100–160°. About 30–45° of arm abduction from the midline is also imparted. The thumb of the hand should be pointing up.

Test contact: With one hand on the distal forearm and the thumb web and thumb of the other hand contacts the lateral edge of and the inferior angle of the scapula.

Patient: Presses the extended arm upwards.

Examiner: Resists the movement of the distal forearm and simultaneously presses the inferior angle of the scapula medially. Weakness is concluded when the humerus descends and the inferior angle of the scapula moves medially almost at the same time. This is a slight improvement of the test as compared those described in the previous literature (Walther 2000, Leaf 1996, Kendall 1983). Classically, muscle weakness was concluded solely by the medial displacement of the inferior angle of the scapula rather than by the combined movement of the arm and scapula together.

Should the inferior angle not move yet the arm descends under resistance pressure, there is a lack of shoulder stabilization. The most frequent cause is weakness of the anterior deltoid.

Test errors, precautions: If movement of the inferior angle of the scapula is not observed, yet the arm descends, differentiation between weakness of the serratus and that of the anterior deltoid cannot be made. Isolating the anterior deltoid and testing it first, will help in the decision-making process. If the anterior deltoid tests strong, the serratus may be assumed to be weak despite the lack of scapular movement. Shortening the lever by moving the contact to a more proximal position (even slightly above the elbow) might be advantageous. In difficult cases, it might be wise to locate and treat all other shoulder muscles first and then return to the serratus anterior.

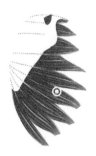

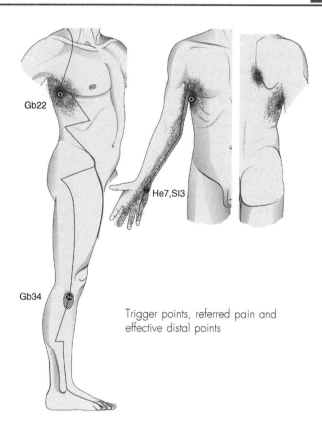

Gb22

He7,SI3

Gb34

Trigger points, referred pain and
effective distal points

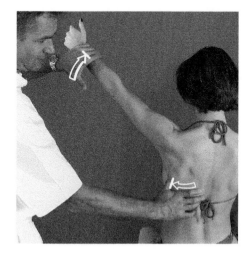

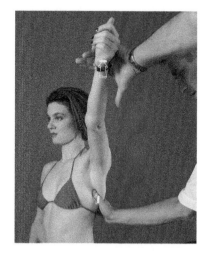

Myofascial syndrome

Stretch test: No stabilization is required if the test is performed in a prone or side-lying position. With the more inferior hand, the examiner contacts the anterior shoulder. The relaxed arm of the patient may lie on the trunk or rest on the forearm of the examiner. The examiner's free hand is moved behind the patient and the fingers curled under the scapula to grasp its medial border. In a coupled movement, both hands are used to synchronously guide the scapula posteriorly and medially while slowly increasing medial rotation of the inferior angle.

PIR: From the stretch position, the patient is asked to press the shoulder forward and elevate the arm. This is performed in several 7–10 s intervals while an inspiration is held. The relaxation phase has the patient slowly breathing out while the examiner gently returns the shoulder and scapula to the stretch position and then slightly beyond.

Frequently found associated disorders

It should be one of the first muscles, besides the subscapularis, to be evaluated when dealing with shoulder problems. It is not uncommon to find a combination of problems ranging from origin-insertion and trigger points to myofascial lesions.

Compression weaknesses: C6 root syndrome from the C5/C6 intervertebral foramen. The long thoracic nerve can be impinged as it passes through the area of the scalenus medius, thus weakening the anterior serratus.

The dorsal scapular nerve may also pass through the scalenus medius and be entrapped there. It innervates the rhomboids and the levator scapula muscles. In the presence of both impingements, a combined pattern of rhomboid, levator scapula and anterior serratus muscle weakness leads to a pronounced instability of the scapula during abduction of the arm.

Motor function innervation: Long thoracic nerve, C5–C7, C(8)
Visceroparietal segment (TS line): T3
Rib pump zone: Intercostal space, costotransverse joint 3, 10
Organ: Lungs
Nutrients: Vitamins C, E, beta carotene, Se, N-acetyl-cysteine
Meridian: Lungs
SRS: Middle thoracic spine; 6th and 7th ribs

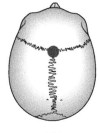

NV

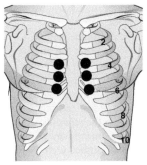

NL anterior

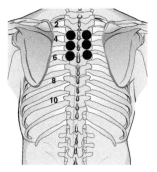

NL posterior

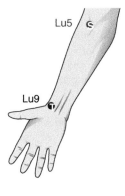

Lu5

Lu9

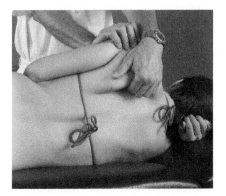

Stretch test and PIR of the serratus anterior

Anatomy

Origin: Dorsal surface of the head of the fibula, proximal third of the fibula, soleal line, middle third of the medial margin of the tibia and the tendinous arch between the head of the fibula and the tibia.

Insertion: Together with the gastrocnemius at the calcaneal tuberosity.

Action

Plantar flexion of the foot at the talocrural (ankle) joint.

Signs of weakness: Forward-leaning posture and inability or instability when attempting to stand on toes.

Test

Position: The patient is placed prone, the knee flexed to 90° and the foot is plantar flexed.

Test contact: Using both hands, one hand is placed on the plantar aspect of the distal forefoot and the other hand grasps the postero-superior part of the calcaneus close to the Achilles tendon insertion.

Examiner: Attempts to push the forefoot down into dorsal extension (towards the table surface) while simultaneously pulling the heel upwards. Note: This is a very difficult movement due to the short lever, strength of the muscle and synergism. The soleus and gastrocnemius are very strong muscles. Despite the disadvantage afforded by the flexed knee position, during the test, they are still working together.

It may be more advantageous for the examiner to use a double hand contact on the forefoot in order to press the foot into dorsal extension. Clinically, only severe weakness of the muscle can be established with this test.

Test errors, precautions: The forefoot should not be too enthusiastically squeezed as this can cause adverse sensory provocation of the metatarsophalangeal joints and false weakness responses. As well pain should not be triggered by the hand that grasps and pulls down on the heel.

Myofascial syndrome

Stretch test: The patient lies prone and flexes the knee fully. Flexion at the knee allows the gastrocnemius to relax and permits an enhanced stretch of the soleus. The examiner, in a coupled movement, pushes the forefoot down into dorsal extension and draws the heel upwards. The directions of movement are the same as those made during the muscle test. During the stretch test, there is no patient resistance to the movement.

PIR: From the stretched position, the patient slowly contracts the muscle by plantar flexing the foot. During the relaxation phase, the examiner gently elongates the muscle by bring the foot back to the stretch position.

Causes for compression: The posterior muscles (tibialis posterior, flexor hallucis longus, flexor hallicus brevis and others may be inhibited, when the soleus is hypertonic, causing an entrapment at the upper margin of the tendinous arch of the soleus.

A Baker's cyst at the posterior knee can lead to compression of the tibial nerve at a point just below the head of the gastrocnemius.

Frequently found associated disorders

Primary hypertonus and contraction are often more common findings with this muscle than weakness. This is especially noted in women who wear high-heeled shoes for lengthy periods of time. Chronic hypertonus and contraction of the muscle can lead to inhibition of the anterior tibialis and, occasionally, the extensor digitorum longus. Eventually, this may lead to the development of a flat foot and calcaneal spurring. Chronic weakness of the muscles in the anterior compartment of the lower leg may self perpetuate the shortening of the triceps surae.

Hypertonus of the soleus may lead to muscle cramping and false claudication-like symptoms, usually caused by a compression of the nerve somewhere between the popliteus and the soleus. Associated muscle weakness is not evident, although plantar paraesthesia is common, especially after activities like jumping or running.

Motor function innervation: Tibial nerve, L5, S1, S2
Rib pump zone: Intercostal space, costotransverse joint 6, 7
Organ: Adrenal gland
Meridian: Pericardium (circulation-sex)
SRS: S1, S3, T12

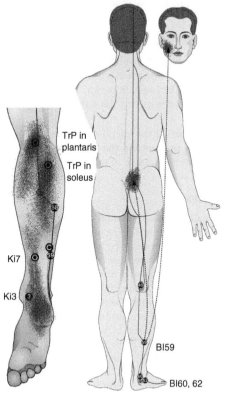

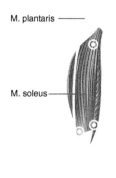

Soleus test

Trigger points in the soleus and plantaris and effective distal points

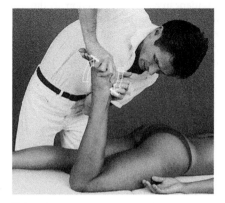

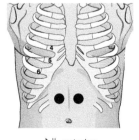

NL anterior

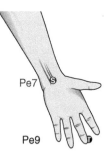

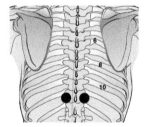

NL posterior

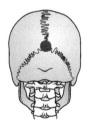

NV

M. sternocleidomastoideus (SCM)

Anatomy

Origin: Sternal head: Superior, anterior surface of the manubrium of the sternum.

Clavicular head: Superior, anterior surface of the medial third of the clavicle.

Insertion: At the lateral surface of the mastoid process and the lateral half of the superior nuchal line of the occiput.

Action

Simultaneous contraction of both sides flexes the cervical spine and, at the endpoint of flexion, the head is extended. The cervical spine flexes in two phases. The first is primarily between the occiput and atlas. The second brings in the rest of the cervical spine. When the cervical spine moves into the second phase of flexion, the angle measured between the C2 and C7 is 45°. At this angle an increased posterior rotation of the occipito-atlantal joints (C0/C1) occurs. It is thought that this mechanism protects the cervical medulla from adverse mechanical insult when a severe hyperflexion trauma is induced into the cervical spine. Hyperflexion-extension (whiplash) trauma would have more severe consequences would it not be for this mechanism. The SCM most likely also aids the nuchal ligament in limiting excessive posterior rotation of these joints.

One-sided contraction rotates the head (face) to the opposite side. The muscle aids in lateral inclination of the cervical spine. If the insertion at the skull is the fixed point, the muscle helps in lifting the upper thorax during forced inspiration.

Note: Cervical spine and head flexion is dependent on the synergistic activity of all the neck muscles – the deep neck flexors, the scalenus muscles and the sternocleidomastoideus.

Signs of weakness: Head rotation to the side of the weakness.

Test

Position: The supine patient's arms are abducted to about 90° and the forearms are flexed at the elbows and rotated backwards. The arm position is supposed to reduce any recruitment from the chest and abdominal muscles. The cervical spine is flexed by lifting the head up as far as possible from the table. The head is then fully rotated so that the nose is on the side opposite to the tested muscle.

The SCM is frequently tested with the patient in a standing position, as the muscle is very sensitive to changes in posture and other afferent stimuli from the periphery. It is one of the most important muscles used in the functional evaluation or receptor changes due to postural alterations.

The cervicodorsal junction must be firmly stabilized for the proper execution of this test. Posterior deviation of the body will cause a reflexive weakness as the brain thinks the body is going to fall over backwards.

Test contact: Over a relatively a broad area on the antero-lateral aspect of the parietal bone. In some, the muscle will weaken suddenly and the head can slam onto the table surface. Therefore, the free hand, without touching, is positioned behind the head to cushion the fall, should a precipitous weakness occur.

Patient: Pushes the head upward (in supine position) or forward and downward (standing or sitting test position) as hard as possible against the testing hand. It is important to make sure that full rotation is maintained during the test. When weak, the natural tendency is to try to rotate the head toward the neutral position, bringing the other neck flexors into the test.

Examiner: Resists in a superior and posterior direction so that the head is extended. The vector direction must strictly follow the tangent of the arc made by the head during flexion.

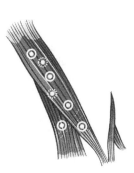

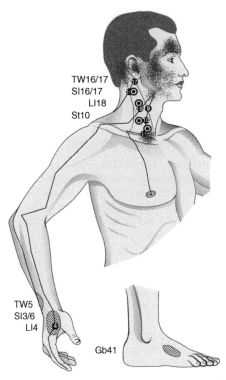

TW16/17
SI16/17
LI18
St10

TW5
SI3/6
LI4

Gb41

Trigger points and effective distal points

Motor function innervation: Accessory nerve (XI), C2 and C3
Organ: Maxillary, frontal sinuses
Nutrients: Vitamin B3, B6, iodine
Meridian: Stomach
SRS: T5–T8

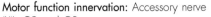

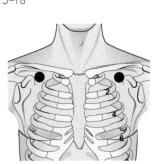

NL anterior

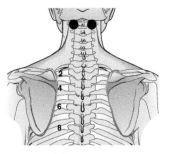

NL posterior

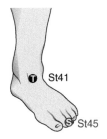

St41

St45

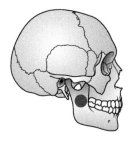

NV

Test errors, precautions: The test resistance vector must be precise otherwise there will be either a false weakness finding or strength in the presence of weakness. Recruitment of the scalenes and other deep neck flexors may negate positive findings. De-rotation of the head during the test must be prevented.

Myofascial syndrome

Stretch test: The head is rotated to the side of the muscle to be stretched and fully extended. Frequently, this movement is restricted due to joint dysfunction in the cervical spine and adverse tension within the muscle itself.

PIR: Starting from the stretch position the patient holds an inspiration for 10 s while gradually lifting the head and simultaneously shifts the eyes to gaze in the direction of the contracting muscle.

At the endpoint of contraction, the patient shifts the gaze back to the other side, and while slowly breathing out, allows the head to descend back down to the table surface.

Frequently found associated disorders

The muscle strongly influences the TMJ and should be examined in any disorder involving the stomatognathic complex. Because the SCM is strongly associated with the cervical spine and the craniomandibular areas it is an ideal indicator muscle for craniomandibular dysfunction (CMD) evaluation. CMD is a complex entity and is always linked to disorders of the upper cervical spine. This is especially noted following whiplash type injuries that cause increased muscle tension and trigger points in the neck and muscles of mastication.

The muscle should be examined and treated as a causal factor in any headache or myofascial pain complaint of the head and neck area.

Compression weakness: Cranial vault and sutural restriction at the base of the skull, including atlanto-occipital joint lesions, can compromise the nerves exiting the jugular foramen. The glossopharangeal, vagus and accessory nerves may be adversely effected.

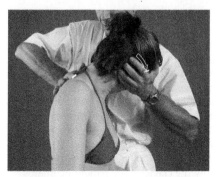

Seated sternocleidomastoid (SCM) test

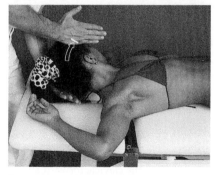

Supine sternocleidomastoid test

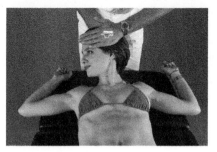

Supine sternocleidomastoid test

Anatomy

Origin: At the superior surface of the first rib and medially as far as the cartilaginous junction.

Insertion: On the undersurface, as far as the centre of the clavicle.

Action

Primarily draws the clavicle forward and down in a slight rotatory fashion. It also minimally assists in flexing and depressing the shoulder. Normal function of the muscle is important for a harmonious rotational movement of the clavicle when lifting the arm above 90°.

Test

All described tests are indirect as the muscle cannot be specifically isolated and are dependent upon the normal function of almost all shoulder muscles. It is recommended that they be evaluated prior to the subclavius.

Position: The arm is extended at the elbow, laterally rotated, abducted and elevated to 180°. The arm should now be alongside the head, almost vertical to the body and with the palm facing medially.

Test contact: On the palmar aspect of the distal forearm.

Stabilization: Superiorly, on the contralateral shoulder.

Patient: Draws the extended arm medially, towards the head and opposite side.

Examiner: Pulls the arm laterally away from the head. Resistance should follow the natural arc of motion described by the arm as it is abducted and elevated into the start position.

The stabilization hand can also be placed over the clavicle in order to palpate it during the test. If increased movement of the clavicle is noted during the test, muscle weakness is indicated.

The test may be performed bilaterally in the same fashion. In this case, both arms are elevated and laterally rotated. The examiner attempts to abduct the arms from the midline simultaneously. Stabilization occurs naturally and is unnecessary.

The classic applied kinesiology indirect test offers another possibility. TL is made with the fingers over the muscle, just below the clavicle. The patient maintains the TL contact and a SIM is tested for weakness. The test should be performed with the arm both in the neutral and elevated positions.

Test errors, precautions: The patient should not be allowed to bend the elbow(s) when testing in the extreme elevated position. Resistance vectors must be strictly maintained.

Myofascial syndrome

Stretch test: No relevant information can be gleaned from a stretch test of the subclavius muscle. Any stretching is hopelessly mingled with that of the clavicular division of the pectoralis major muscle.

PIR: Is not relevant here and omitted. Treatment is made exclusively through the use of deep massage such as fascial flushing, trigger point injection or dry needling.

Cause for compression: The subclavius is involved in costoclavicular compression syndrome. Hypertonus of the muscle can lead to additional closure of the costoclavicular passage and subsequent compression of the nerves of the brachial plexus.

Frequently found associated disorders

The muscle must be considered in any shoulder complaint.

Compression weakness: C5 root lesion. Scalenus syndrome.

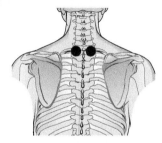

NL posterior

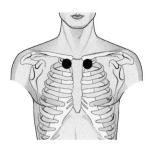

NL anterior

Motor function innervation:
Subclavian nerve, C4, C5, C6
Nutrients: Magnesium

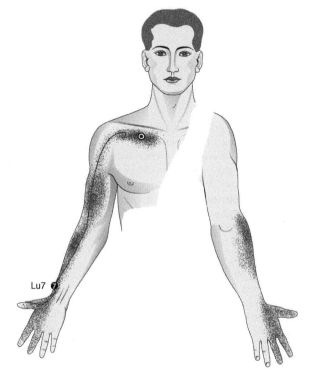

Lu7

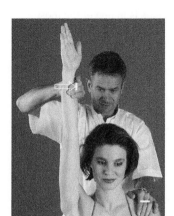

Subclavius: Beardall test

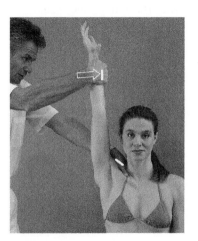

Palpating clavicular movement during the test may be useful

Anatomy

Origin: From almost the entire subscapular fossa or anterior surface (underside) of the scapula.

Course: From the broad insertion it converges anteriorly and laterally and near the medial border of the scapula the serratus anterior passes over and cover it anteriorly.

Insertion: Minor tubercle of the humerus and inferior part of the shoulder joint capsule.

Action

Medial rotation and adduction of the humerus. As one of the rotator cuff muscles, it is the primary anterior stabilizer of the head of the humerus in the glenoid cavity during abduction.

Signs of weaknes: Lateral rotation of the arm when standing so that the palm of the hand points anteriorly.

Test

Position: The elbow is flexed to 90° and the humerus is normally abducted about 90° and then fully medially rotated. Abduction of the humerus to less than 90° will tend to isolate the more superior fibres and with a full abduction of 90° the fibres more inferiorly placed are tested.

Test contact: On the palmar surface of the distal forearm. The testing hand should avoid contacting the acupuncture drainage point He7 in the area of the pisiform bone.

Stabilization: On the radial side of the elbow.

Patient: Keeping the elbow abducted, pushes the hand downward to medially rotate the arm as far as possible. As with several other muscle tests, it might be wise to have a 'dry run or rehearsal' prior to the actual testing.

Examiner: Attempts to laterally rotate the humerus by resisting the downward motion of the patient's hand.

Test errors, precautions: Too little medial rotation of the humerus may lead to a false test. Inadequate stabilization at the elbow, that allows to abduct and/or elevate the shoulder on behalf of the patient are common. Both lead to false interpretation of the test due to synergistic muscle recruitment. In difficult cases an alternative stabilization may be used, whereby the stabilizing hand grasps the patient's shoulder so that the forearm forms a bridge upon which the patient's arm and elbow may rest. The idea is similar to that of the supine quadriceps test. The arm and elbow of the patient are now locked into the testing position. The patient fully rotates the humerus medially and resistance by the examiner is as described above.

Myofascial syndrome

Stretch test: The upper arm is abducted 90° and rotated laterally as far as it will naturally go.

PIR: From the stretch position, the patient slowly rotates the arm into medially. The relaxation phase elongates the muscle by the examiner laterally rotating the arm to gently bring it back to the start position.

Frequently found associated disorders

The subscapularis is in one of the most commonly found muscles involved in functional disorders of the shoulder. It has a similar frequency of involvement to that of the anterior serratus. Hypertonic contraction of the subscapularis is often noted in conjunction with weakness of the antagonistic lateral rotators, particularly the infraspinatus.

The subscapularis should always be considered involved in any case of adhesive capsulitis (frozen shoulder).

Compression weakness: C6 root lesion, scalenus syndrome.

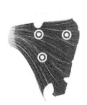

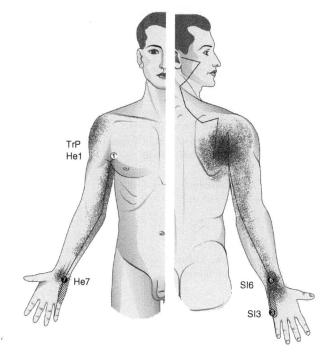

TrP
He1

He7

SI6

SI3

Motor function innervation:
Subscapular nerve, C5, C6 (C7)
Visceroparietal segment (TS line): T2
Rib pump zone: Intercostal space, costotransverse joint 1, 2, 6, 10
Organ: Heart
Nutrients: Vitamins E, B2 and B3, magnesium, carnitine
Meridian: Heart

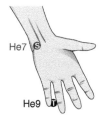

He7

He9

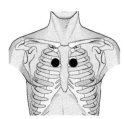

NL anterior

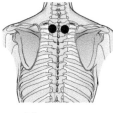

NL posterior

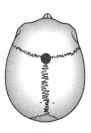

NV

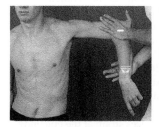

Subscapularis test. Reducing elbow abduction to 45–60° will test the more superior fibres

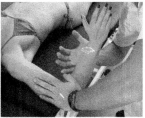

Subscapularis test in the supine position. Avoid touching the He7 drainage point

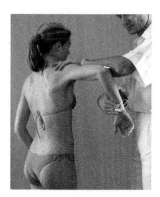

Alternative test position for the subscapularis

Anatomy

Origin: On the lateral epicondyle of the humerus, the dorsal surface of the ulna (crest of the supinatoris ulnae), the lateral collateral ligament of the elbow joint and the annular ligament of the radius.

Course: From proximal to distal in a spiral fashion and around the radius to its insertion.

Insertion: On the proximal third of the volar surface of the radius.

Action

Supinates the forearm.

Signs of weakness: The arm may hang with the hand in pronation.

Test

Position: The forearm is supinated and the shoulder and elbow are fully flexed to reduce the strong supination effect of the biceps.

Stabilization: At the elbow, if not using a double hand contact for better resistance.

Test contact: Around the distal forearm with one hand or both hands with clasped fingers.

Patient: Attempts to keep the forearm in supination.

Examiner: Resists trying to pronate the wrist.

Alternative tests

Position: The forearm is fully supinated, the elbow fully extended, and the arm extended behind the back to about 45°. The hand will end up behind the back with the palm facing the floor. With the elbow and arm in extension, the ability of the biceps to supinate the forearm is almost totally eliminated. In this position, the action of the biceps will be limited to flexing the humerus at the shoulder.

Stabilization: At the elbow if needed.

Test contact: Broadly around the distal forearm.

Patient: Attempts to keep the arm supinated.

Examiner: Resists trying to pronate the wrist.

Test errors: No pain should be caused at the wrist and any rotation, abduction and/or adduction of the humerus should be prevented.

Myofascial syndrome

Stretch test: The elbow is extended and the forearm pronated as far as it will go. Medial rotation of the humerus should not be allowed.

PIR: The elbow is supported by the hand of the examiner and extended. This is followed by full pronation of the forearm. A slow contraction to supinate the forearm is made by the patient against a gentle resistance by the examiner. For the relaxation phase, a gradual elongation of the muscle is introduced by returning it to the stretch position.

Causes for compression: If hypertonicity is present, a 'supinator syndrome' may develop whereby the supinator muscle compromises the deep branch of the radial nerve. This leads to weakness of the muscles innervated by the nerve distal to the entrapment: the extensor digitorum, extensor carpi ulnaris, abductor pollicis longus, extensor pollicis longus and brevis, and extensor indicis.

Frequently found associated disorders

'Tennis elbow' may be a sequel to long-term weakness of the muscle due to lack of stabilization at the proximal radioulnar articulation. Although tennis elbow is not a problem solely associated with tennis, it is important during play to keep the elbow slightly bent. This is especially true for the backhand stroke. Ulnar adduction of the hand on the wrist should be avoided as well. Both situations put undue stress on the forearm at the end of the stroke. As a result, the supinator can eventually weaken. An 'epicondyle clasp', with a cushion in the area of the bellies of the supinator, brachioradialis and extensor carpi radialis, can be worn when playing. Wrapped around the forearm, the cushion places pressure on the muscles and reduces strain at the epicondylar area. For best results it is important to position the clasp correctly, always remembering that it is a crutch, not a cure.

Compression weakness: C6 root lesion, thoracic inlet and radial nerve sulcus syndrome.

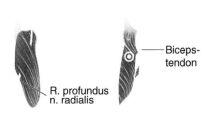

Biceps-
tendon

R. profundus
n. radialis

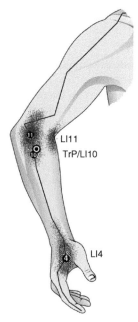

LI11

TrP/LI10

LI4

Trigger points and effective distal points

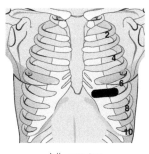

NL anterior

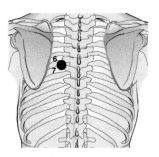

NL posterior

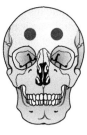

NV

Motor function innervation: Radial nerve, C5, C6 (C7)
Organ: Stomach
Nutrients: Ca, Mg, Fe, phosphatase, Vitamin B5, PUFA
Meridian: Stomach

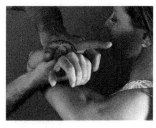

Supinator test

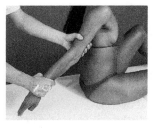

Supinator test

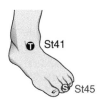

St41

St45

Anatomy

Origin: Medial two-thirds of the supraspinatus fossa.

Course: Laterally from the origin passing under the acromion to the head of the humerus. The bony acromion and subacromial bursa keep the tendon in place.

Insertion: At the upper part of the major tubercle and the joint capsule.

Action

Abduction of the humerus. The muscle is the main mover until about 20–30° of abduction. With the arm at rest, the muscle evidences a constant tone that is believed to aid in keeping the head of the humerus within the shallow glenoid cavity. Its tendon spans the superior joint capsule, but remains extracapsular.

Signs of weakness: With more severe weakness, initial abduction of the arm can only be made by bringing the arm to a point whereby the deltoid muscle may take over. Several classic methods are used. The first is made by laterally bending the body towards the side of weakness so that the arm hangs more perpendicular to the shoulder. The second is seen as a sharp 'flicking' of the arm laterally by the hip or the opposite hand. Normally, it is only with extreme weakness that this becomes necessary. Functional weakness is more common and will create a gradual onset of pain due to compromised joint stability. Weakness predisposes the individual to greater trauma should the need arise to use the arm in a forceful situation, such as to break a fall.

Test

Position: The arm is extended at the elbow and abducted about 15–25°. The arm should be kept in a neutral position without rotation.

Test contact: On the distal forearm.

Stabilization: Is usually not needed, but the free hand can be placed over the acromioclavicular joint and the scapula in order to feel for muscle contraction.

If necessary, when performing the test standing or sitting, the contralateral shoulder may be stabilized.

Patient: Presses the extended arm laterally away from the body.

Examiner: Resists by pushing the arm into adduction in a direction that is more or less towards the greater trochanter of the femur.

Test errors, precautions: The patient must neither bend the elbow nor be allowed to incline the upper body to the tested side. This will change the abduction angle and permit the patient to recruit the deltoids.

Myofascial syndrome

Stretch test: With the arm medially rotated and adducted the patient reaches for the opposite shoulder blade.

PIR: From the stretch position the patient slowly pulls the arm into abduction. This is followed by the relaxation phase where the examiner elongates the muscle by guiding the arm back to the start position.

Frequently found associated disorders

Supraspinatus tendinosis or 'painful arc' syndrome. Painful arc describes the pain felt when the arm is abducted. The pain peaks in the mid-phase of the movement and is usually associated with supraspinatus tendinitis. There may also be other causes of painful arc. The supraspinatus is frequently linked to imbalances of the other muscles of the rotator cuff.

Compression weakness: A lesion of the C5 root leads to weakness of the supraspinatus and all the other shoulder abductors. The suprascapular nerve may become entrapped as it passes through the foramen made by the suprascapular notch below and the transverse scapular ligament above causing suprascapular nerve syndrome. Disharmony between the serratus anterior and rhomboid muscles is the most common cause of entrapment and usually affects the infraspinatus first.

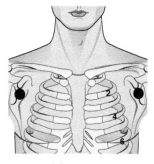

NL anterior

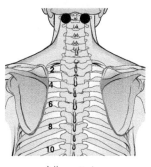

NL posterior

Motor function innervation: Subscapular nerve, C4, C5, C6

Rib pump zone: Intercostal space, costotransverse joint 1, 11

Organ: Brain, pituitary oesophagus

Nutrients: PUFA, antioxidants, choline

Meridian: Conception vessel

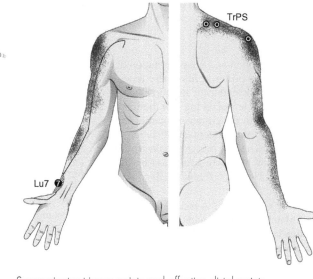

Supraspinatus trigger points and effective distal points

NV

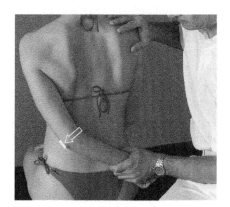

PIR: contraction phase

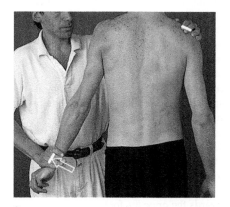

Supraspinatus test

Anatomy

Origin: From the lateral aspect of the superior anterior iliac spine and the anterior part of the iliac crest.

Course: Merges inferiorly into the iliotibial tract of the fascia lata at the transition from the proximal to the middle third of the thigh.

Insertion: The anterior fibres insert into the lateral retinaculum of the patella and the patellar ligament. The posterior fibres insert via the iliotibial tract at the lateral tubercle of the tibia.

Action

Flexion, abduction and medial rotation of the femur. The posterior fibres also have some effect in keeping the knee in extension. The muscle inserts into the iliotibial tract along with the gluteus maximus and together they aid in lateral stabilization of the knee. The two muscles make up 'the deltoid of the hip', acting on it as does the deltoid muscle in the shoulder (Kapandji 2001).

Signs of weakness: A lack of lateral knee stability during flexion and in some circumstances genu varum. An aching sensation at the anterior hip, close to the insertion of the muscle.

Test

Position: The test is performed in the supine position. The leg is fully rotated medially and extended at the knee. It is abducted and flexed at the hip in both directions to about 30°.

Test contact: On the lateral aspect of the distal part of the leg, close to the lateral malleolus.

Stabilization: On the distal and lateral aspect of the contralateral leg close to or on the lateral malleolus.

Patient: Presses the extended leg outwards and slightly upwards in a diagonal direction of abduction.

Examiner: Resists the diagonal motion in a direction that would bring the leg towards the opposite foot.

Test errors, precautions: The patient must precisely follow the diagonal (out and up) directional movement of the leg. All of the following must not be permitted: A straight elevation, linear abduction or external rotation of the leg, as well as, any knee flexion. As with the psoas test, the extended leg should be initially supported to prevent fatiguing the muscle. As soon as the examiner notes correct directional movement, the testing hand should be opened so that there is only a flat contact made by the palm. Thus, the examiner can more easily sense subtle changes in the resistance direction and not over-power the patient with too much pressure. The examiner must be vigilant in following the resistance vector towards the opposite foot. Any deviation will tend to invalidate the test.

Myofascial syndrome

Stretch test: The patient is placed in a side-lying position with the back close to the edge of the table. The lower leg is bent and rests on the table surface to prevent trunk rotation. The frontal plane of the pelvis is rotated a bit forward so that it forms about a 45° angle to the table surface. The examiner, standing behind, makes body contact on the posterior trunk or pelvis of the patient to help in stabilizing the pelvis during the procedure. The superior leg is guided into extension, adduction and lateral rotation by bringing it backward and downward over the edge of the table.

PIR: From the position of stretch and with a sustained inspiration, the extended leg is slowly abducted, flexed and medially rotated so that it arrives more or less in the original test position described above. During a prolonged expiration the extended leg is again brought back to the stretch position. Elongation is made solely by the weight of the leg.

Frequently found associated disorders

Lateral thigh pain, lateral knee pain and pelvic lesions. Iron-deficiency anaemia has been related to bilateral functional weakness of the muscle, but this has yet to be confirmed.

Compression weakness: L4 and L5 root lesions, piriformis syndrome (compression of the superior gluteal nerve (n. gluteus sup) as it passes through the suprapiriform foramen).

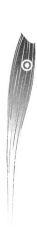
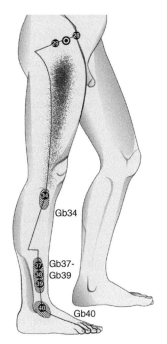
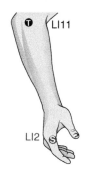

Gb34

Gb37-
Gb39

Gb40

Trigger points and effective distal points

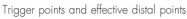

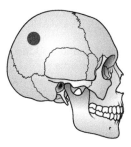

NV

Motor function innervation: Superior gluteal nerve,
L4, L5 and S1
Organ: Large intestine
Nutrients: Iron (for bilateral functional weakness),
intestinal symbionts (lactobacillus, E. coli), l-glutamine
Meridian: Large intestine
SRS: L3
Rib pump zone: Intercostal space,
costotransverse joint 3, 10

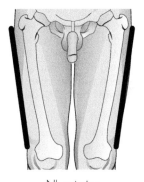

NL anterior

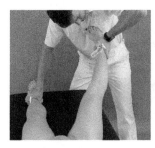

Tensor fasciae latae test

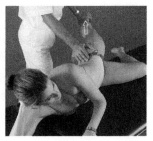

PIR of the tensor fasciae lata:
contraction phase

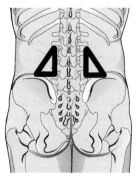

NL posterior

Anatomy

Origin: At the dorsal surface of the scapula in the area of the inferior angle and the caudal third of the lateral margin of the scapula.

Course: Laterally and superiorly to the anterior aspect of the humerus.

Insertion: At the minor tubercle (medial lip of the bicipital groove) of the humerus blending with the fibres of the latissimus dorsi.

Action

Medial rotation, adduction and extension of the humerus.

Signs of weakness: Rarely, an increased lateral rotation of the arm when standing.

Test

Position: Independent of patient position, the elbow is flexed to 90° and the humerus put in full medial rotation. The hand is made into a fist to reinforce the wrist and reduce any possibility of TL. The fist is then placed on the posterior part of the iliac crest, close to the SI joint. This position puts the humerus in maximum extension with the elbow projecting backwards from the posterior trunk.

One-sided test

Note that all teres major tests are extremely difficult to evaluate due to the strong synergistic activity of the latissimus dorsi muscle.

Position: Performed while sitting or, if necessary, standing. In order to extract the latissimus dorsi from the test, the elbow must be brought as far backward toward the dorsal spine as is physically possible.

Test contact: On the medial aspect of the elbow.

Stabilization: The patient's trunk and shoulder are stabilized with the non-testing hand and the examiner's own body (chest).

Bilateral test

Position: Best performed with the patient prone as the table surface offers a firm stabilization. Resistance is made on both elbows simultaneously and this manoeuvre, along with the body weight in the prone position has a stabilizing effect during the test. Some examiners prefer to cross the testing arms to improve the inward-outward vector of resistance.

Patient: Presses the elbows together and back as strongly as is possible. The start position should begin with the elbows as far towards the midline as is possible. Individuals with very strong and/or shortened pectoral muscles may have difficulty approximating the elbows and the latissimus dorsi will remain active during the test.

Examiner: Resists first by attempting to separate the elbows from one another and then, if lateral movement ensues, follows the arc of motion described by the elbow as it abducts from the midline.

Test errors, precautions: Too little extension and adduction of the humerus and contact pain at the elbow. The examiner must be very aware of latissimus dorsi recruitment patterns by the patient. A few degrees of abduction from the midline by the elbows will bring the latissimus muscle strongly into the test. (Recall the body-builder posture for demonstrating the latissimus muscle.) Too slow resistance or lack of continued resistance will allow the latissimus to be recruited as well.

Myofascial syndrome

Stretch test: The arm is guided behind the head to put it into abduction and lateral rotation.

PIR: From the stretch position and with a sustained inspiration, the patient gradually brings the arm and elbow down into adduction. In the relaxation phase, the patient breathes out slowly as the examiner gently elongates the muscle by returning the limb to the stretch position.

Frequently found associated disorders

Bilateral functional weakness indicates possible micro-fixations of the thoracic spine.

Compression weakness: C6 root lesion, scalenus syndrome.

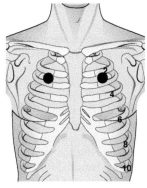

NL anterior

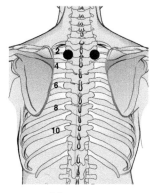

NL posterior

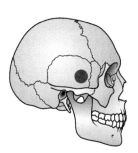

NV

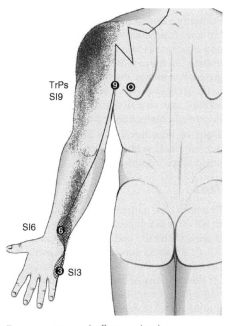

Motor function innervation:
N. thoracodorsalis, C5, C6, C7
Organ: Vertebral column
Nutrients: Substances that regulate the acid–base balance (Leaf, 1996), zinc
Meridian: Governing vessel, Du Mai
Rib pump zone: intercostal space, costotransverse joint 9

Trigger points and effective distal points

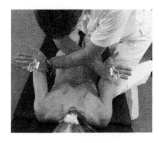

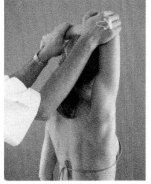

PIR of the teres major

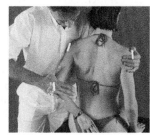

Teres major test – bilateral and unilateral

Anatomy

Origin: On the dorsal surface of the scapula along the middle third of its lateral margin. It also arises from two aponeurotic laminae that separate it from the infraspinatus and teres major muscles.

Course: In an oblique direction laterally and superiorly.

Insertion: In the most inferior depression of the greater tubercle of the humerus and slightly below the articular capsule.

Action

Primarily a lateral rotation of the humerus, but a weak accessory effect of adduction and extension is also imparted by the muscle. Along with the other rotary cuff group, it stabilizes the head of the humerus in the glenoid cavity. This stabilizing activity continues dynamically during flexion and abduction of the humerus.

Signs of weakness: An increased internal rotation of the arm that is best noted when standing.

Test

Position: The patient's elbow is flexed to 90°. This is followed by rotating the humerus laterally and then abducted about 20°. A 20° abduction brings the humerus to the best angle that aligns the muscle fibres for the test. Any abduction more than 20° will tend to bring the infraspinatus muscle into the test. The forearm is kept in a neutral position so that the thumb is uppermost.

Test contact: On the dorsal aspect of the distal forearm. Due to the position of the forearm the contact will naturally be lateral to the midline of the body.

Stabilization: The free hand stabilizes the elbow medially, avoiding the drainage point TH 10. The point is located in a depression found about one human inch (the thumb's width of an individual) above the olecranon process.

Patient: Presses the wrist outward so as to laterally rotate the humerus.

Examiner: Resists by pushing the wrist toward the midline to medially rotate the arm.

Test errors, precautions: Should external rotation be reduced, the other shoulder fixators will be allowed to lock the shoulder down. Attempts by the patient to abduct the arm, instead of laterally rotating, and too much abduction at the start of the test (greater than 20–30°), leads to excessive recruitment of the infraspinatus. The elbow must be securely fixed in place.

Myofascial syndrome

Stretch test: The arm is flexed (the degree is not important) at the elbow. This is followed by abduction and medial rotation of the humerus, so that the elbow is elevated at least 90° from the trunk. The teres major, infraspinatus and latissimus dorsi muscles are, to some extent, also stretched. Differentiation between the muscles is achieved by palpation over the muscles or by performing the 'hand to shoulder blade' test. If the patient cannot manage to reach behind the back and touch the opposite scapula, shortening of the lateral rotators (teres minor and infraspinatus) is present. Normally, in these cases, the patient will not be able to place the hand much farther than the hip or SI joint.

PIR: From the stretch position and with a sustained inspiration, the patient slowly moves the elbow down and the wrist up to bring the humerus into adduction and lateral rotation. During expiration the examiner gently elongates the muscle by returning the limb to the stretch position.

Frequently found associated disorders

Thyroid disorders and shoulder problems.

Compression weakness: C5 or C6 root lesion, scalenus syndrome, costoclavicular syndrome, pectoralis minor syndrome.

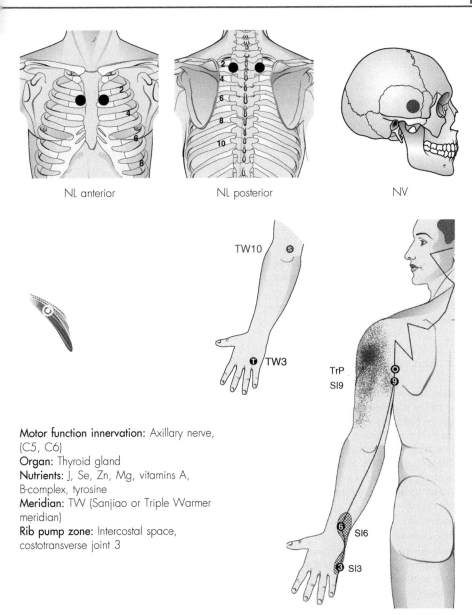

NL anterior   NL posterior   NV

TW10

TW3

TrP
SI9

9

SI6

SI3

Motor function innervation: Axillary nerve, (C5, C6)
Organ: Thyroid gland
Nutrients: J, Se, Zn, Mg, vitamins A, B-complex, tyrosine
Meridian: TW (Sanjiao or Triple Warmer meridian)
Rib pump zone: Intercostal space, costotransverse joint 3

Trigger points and effective distal points

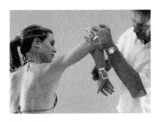
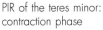
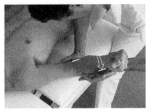

PIR of the teres minor: contraction phase

Teres minor test

Anatomy

Origin: At the lateral condyle and upper two-thirds of the lateral surface of the tibia, the interosseous membrane and the fascia cruris.

Course: Running from superior to inferior, it is the most medial and anterior muscle of the anterior (fibular) compartment.

Insertion: At the medial and plantar surface of the medial cuneiform bone and the base of the 1st metatarsal.

Action

Strongly dorsiflexes the foot primarily at the talocrural joint and inverts the foot at the subtalar and tarsal joints.

Signs of weakness: Flat footedness and, in severe weakness, foot drop.

Test

Note: Hand positions are reversed for the left side.

Position (right side): Standing or sitting at the feet of the patient, the examiner grasps the right foot with the right hand and turns it into supination. The palm will be contacting the bottom and the fingers the dorsum of the foot. Maintaining supination, the foot is put into full extension, trying, as well. to keep the big toe flexed.

Stabilization: The free hand firmly grasps the heel from underneath.

Patient: Keeping the foot supinated, draws the forefoot up towards the head as strongly as possible.

Examiner: Resists into plantarflexion by pulling strongly downward on the foot.

Alternative test

Test contact (right side): The contact changes such that the foot is grasped from above so that the thumb is now on the dorsum and the fingers on the plantar aspect of the foot. The examiner's elbow is moved superiorly, automatically supinating the foot and aligning the arm to follow the proper resistance vector. Dorsiflexion completes the positioning.

Stabilization: The free hand firmly stabilizes the heel, especially laterally, from below.

Patient: Maintaining supination, draws the forefoot towards the head in the direction of dorsiflexion.

Examiner: Resists in a direction of plantar flexion and, as the foot begins to descend, also following the arc of motion as the foot everts.

Test errors, precautions: The position and the vector of the test must be adhered to with strict precision. No contact made by the testing or the stabilizing hand should provoke pain. This is especially important when bunions are present and limits the ability of the examiner to keep the big toe flexed during the test.

Myofascial syndrome

Stretch test: The foot is placed in plantar flexion and eversion (pronation).

PIR: Starting from the stretch position, the patient pulls the foot into dorsiflexion and inversion (supination) against resistance by the examiner. In the relaxation phase the examiner brings the foot back to the stretch position.

Frequently found associated disorders

A hypertonic tibialis anterior can lead to reflex inhibition of the psoas and the vastus divisions of the quadriceps. Compensatory gait disorders, like a shortened stride, will result. Hypertonicity and contraction of the gastrocnemius and soleus muscles (triceps surae) can lead to reflex inhibition of the tibialis anterior. Conversely, a weak tibialis anterior can lead to reflex contraction and hypertonicity of the triceps surae.

Compression weakness: Piriformis and fibular tunnel syndromes. According to Patten 1998 and Walther 2000, it is the indicator muscle for L4 root (L3/4 disc); others include the L5 root.

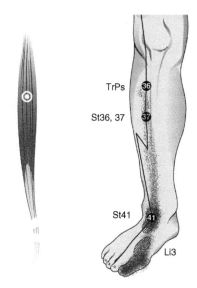

TrPs

St36, 37

St41

Li3

Trigger points and
effective distal points

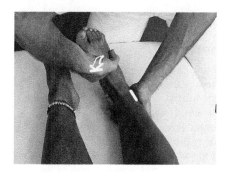

Alternative test position

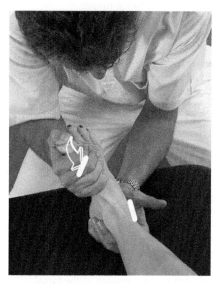

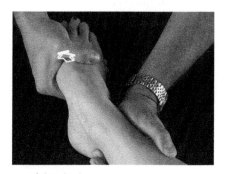

PIR of the tibialis anterior

Tibialis anterior test: the big toe is held in
flexion to avoid extensor hallucis muscle
recruitment

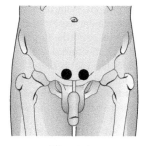

NL anterior

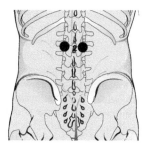

NL posterior

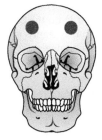

NV

Motor function innervation: Deep fibular nerve, L4, L5 and S1
Organ: Bladder
Nutrients: Vitamin A, vitamin B complex, potassium
Meridian: Bladder
SRS: L4
Rib pump zone: Intercostal space, costotransverse joint 6, 8

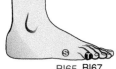

Bl65 Bl67

Anatomy

Origin: On the lateral part of the dorsal surface of the tibia, the proximal two-thirds of the medial surface of the fibula and the interosseous membrane.

Course: From superior to inferior in the same plane as the flexor hallucis longus and flexor digitorum longus in the deep layer of the dorsal muscle group of the lower leg. All of the tendons of the three muscles pass behind the medial malleolus and through the tarsal tunnel.

Insertion: In a splayed fashion on the plantar aspect of the foot covering an area from the tuberosity of navicular, the medial cuneiform, cuboid and the bases of the 2nd to 4th metatarsal bones. There are also recurrent stretches of tendon to the sustentaculum tali of the calcaneus.

Action

Inverts and plantar flexes the foot and provides dynamic support for the medial arch of the foot.

Signs of weakness: Posterior tibial tendon dysfunction (PTTD) and adult acquired flat footedness are common. Other consequences of weakness may occur as well, like difficulty walking on the toes and weakness of the flexor hallucis brevis due to compression at the tarsal tunnel when the body weight is on the foot.

Test

Position: With the patient supine, the examiner stands at the foot of the examining table.

Test contact (right tibialis posterior): There are several possible contacts for this test and the examiner should decide which is best. With the right hand the examiner grasps the medial aspect of the distal foot so that the thumb is on the dorsum and the fingers on the plantar aspect. The web between the thumb and index finger should now be in contact with the distal,

medial forefoot close to the proximal joint of the big toe. When satisfied with the contact, the foot is brought down into full plantar flexion and slight inversion. The amount of plantar flexion and inversion will differ significantly between patients. With the foot in the test position, the elbow of the testing hand must be brought down so that the forearm is at the same level of the plantar flexed foot.

Stabilization: Under the heel with the free (left) hand and covering the lateral calcaneus.

Patient: Pushes the foot down into plantar flexion and inwards into adduction.

Examiner: Resists at the start of the test from medial to lateral. When the forefoot begins to move, the examiner continues the resistance following the arc of motion of dorsiflexion and eversion. Examiner resistance should strictly adhere to the vector made by the forefoot in achieving this position.

Hand positioning is reversed for the left tibialis posterior.

During the test it is critical to carefully observe for tibialis anterior muscle recruitment. Contraction of the muscle will elevate the tendon against the anterior tensor retinaculum and is an easily visible sign of recruitment during testing.

Alternative test (right tibialis posterior)

Test contact: Standing at the foot of the table, the examiner takes a position to the lateral side of the right foot. With the palm of the right hand, the plantar aspect of the foot is contacted. At this point the fingers curl up and over the medial and dorsal aspects of the big toe. The foot is then plantar flexed and inverted, taking care not to allow any tibial rotation. The examiner's elbow should be down, parallel to the table surface.

Stabilization: The heel of the foot is placed in the cupped left hand with the calcaneus stabilized laterally by the base of the palm.

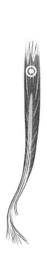

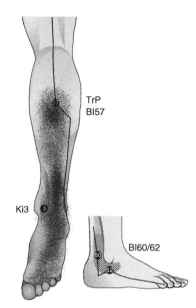

TrP
Bl57

Ki3

Bl60/62

Trigger points and effective distal points

Motor function innervation: Tibial nerve, L4, L5 and S1
Organ: Adrenal gland
Nutrients: Tyrosine and other cofactors of catecholamine synthesis: vitamins B3, B6, B12 and folic acid; vitamin B5, vitamin C, manganese, ginseng
Meridian: Pericardium (circulation-sex)
SRS: L1, L5, S1
Rib pump zone: Intercostal space, costotransverse joint 3, 8

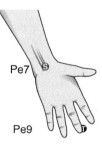

Pe7

Pe9

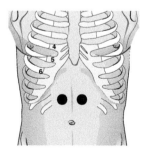

NL anterior

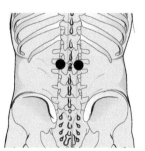

NL posterior

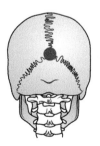

NV

Patient: Pushes the foot medially, with plantar flexion strictly maintained. As described above, all the resistance vectors must be precisely followed.

Hand positioning is reversed for the left foot.

Test errors, precautions: It is a particularly difficult muscle to isolate. The lever is very short and with incremental changes in leg and foot position the tibialis anterior will enter into the test. Too little plantar flexion leads to massive recruitment of the tibialis anterior and should be avoided at all costs. The contacts made by the testing and stabilizing hand should not be painful. Avoid any medial rotation of the tibia during the test. Medial rotation is an indication of weakness and will change the testing vector allowing the tibialis anterior to become involved.

Myofascial syndrome

Stretch test: Pronate (evert) and dorsiflex (extend) the foot.

PIR: Starting from the stretch position the patient slowly brings the foot into inversion and plantar flexion against a gentle resistance from the examiner. In the relaxation phase, the examiner elongates the muscle by, gradually, returning the foot to the stretch position.

Frequently found associated disorders

Fallen arches, plantar and tarsal tunnel pain in the push-off phase of gait. Over pronation of the foot may develop and is a weakness frequently related to chronic hypoadrenia. In children having suffered from intrauterine stress syndrome, bilateral weakness is often found together with a host of secondary foot disorders. As the infant is not yet ambulatory, the problem is usually not immediately evident and only begins to evolve when walking commences.

A palpatory pain pattern, associated with chronic tibialis posterior weakness has been reported by Leaf (1996). He found a high correlation between tibialis posterior muscle weakness and ipsilateral palpatory pain at the lateral calcaneus, medial knee, greater trochanter and in the following muscles: lumbar spinal extensors, rhomboids, scalenus anterior and pterygoids.

Compression weakness: Compression of the tibial nerve with iliolumbar ligament syndrome, piriformis syndrome and popliteus syndrome. According to Patten (1998) a lesion of the S1 root, from the L5/ S1 disc, will cause weakness of both the tibialis posterior and the gastrocnemius muscles.

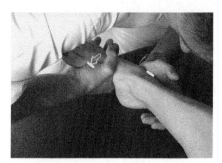

Tibialis posterior test

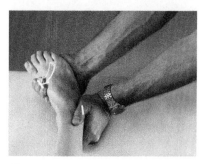

Alternative test position

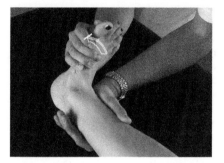

PIR of the tibialis posterior

M. trapezius (pars inferior, pars ascendens)

Anatomy

Origin: On the spinous processes of T6 to T12.

Course: The most superficial of the back muscles, the fibres run laterally and superiorly, converging fan shape.

Insertion: At the medial third of the spine of the scapula.

Action

Retraction and depression of the scapula, but also a rotation of the scapula, so that the glenoid cavity rotates upward (cranially). The medial border will be drawn downward and towards the vertebral column. Along with other muscles, it helps to keep the spine in an upright, extended position.

Signs of weakness: When standing, the shoulder will appear higher than normal, coupled with an increased forward flexion type posture. An increased kyphosis of the thoracic spine with a classic 'rounded back' is evident in patients with a chronic, bilateral weakness of the muscles.

Test

Position: The classic test is made with the patient prone and the side to be tested close to the edge of the table. The arm is extended at the elbow, abducted to about 130° and laterally rotated so that the thumb points backwards. The thumb will be seen by the examiner to be pointing upwards, away from the floor. The head can be rotated to the side of the test in order to take out any synergism of the upper trapezius.

Test contact: With a light contact allowing more sensitivity due to the long lever and relative weakness of the muscle. As few as two or three fingers may be used to increase examiner sensitivity.

Stabilization: On the posterior thorax in order to restrict any body rotation that might occur.

Patient: Presses the extended arm back-wards and upwards (dorsally). The movement is very difficult for most patients and the amount of strength generated not great.

Examiner: Resists by pushing the arm lightly downward in an anterior direction.

It must be remembered that this is an indirect muscle test. Since the muscle does not insert on the humerus, a descent of the arm during the test, is not a conclusive indication of muscle weakness. The ability of the patient to keep the inferior angle of the scapula from moving is the crucial factor in determining a weakness. If no movement of the inferior angle of the scapula is noted, yet the arm moves anteriorly towards the floor, the indication is that most likely the trapezius is functioning normally. The probable cause is a weakness of the muscles fixating the posterior the shoulder, especially the posterior deltoid.

The test can also be carried out in the supine position where stabilization of the patient is generally better but palpation of the inferior angle of the scapula is made more difficult. One should be aware that both Kendall and Walther report that testing in the supine position may lead to a false finding. In the supine position, the scapula is fixed against the table surface by the weight of the body.

The muscle may be tested with the patient sitting or standing. In theses cases, stabilization of the anterior shoulder on the tested side is necessary.

Test errors, precautions: The test must be carried out very carefully, as the lever is very long compared to the strength of the muscle in the average patient. When weakness is indicated, it is best to evaluate both the posterior division of the deltoid and the lower trapezius. Only when the posterior deltoid is tested strong can a specific differential diagnosis be made for the inferior trapezius.

Myofascial syndrome

Stretch test: Specific stretch testing is not possible. With the trunk and shoulders of the seated patient rolled forward the muscle may be palpated for trigger points and referred pain provocation.

Frequently found associated disorders

Recurrent rib lesions are common and with bilateral weakness, micro-fixations of the thoracolumbar vertebrae are regularly found. When weakness is chronic an increased thoracic kyphosis often develops.

Compression weakness: Mechanical lesions of the third and fourth cervical vertebrae as well as any dysfunction around the base of the skull that adversely influences the accessory nerve as it exits from the jugular foramen. Compromise of the accessory nerve will primarily affect the upper trapezius.

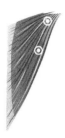

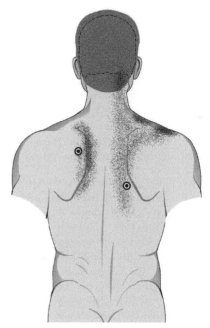

Trigger points and referred pain patterns. Note: The upper trigger point shown in the left illustration in this figure is depicted on the left side, the lower one on the right.

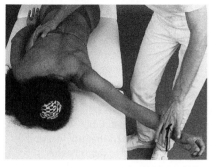

Test of the ascending fibres. The stabilizing hand may also be placed on the scapula on the tested side. Note: this makes the stabilization less sure

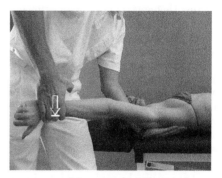

Supine test of the ascending fibres with simultaneous palpation of the scapula

Anatomy

Origin: From the spinal processes of T1 to T5.

Course: Muscle fibres run laterally and horizontally.

Insertion: At the spine of the scapula and the posterior acromion.

Action

Retracts and partially assists in the elevation of the scapula. When the scapula is fixed, it aids in retracting the shoulder.

Signs of weakness: Protraction of the shoulder and a rounded back.

Test

Position: In the classic test, like that of the inferior trapezius, the patient lies prone. The arm is extended at the elbow, abducted to 90° and fully laterally rotated so that the thumb points backwards, away from the floor. To the examiner this will appear to be upwards.

Test contact: On the distal aspect of the radial bone of the fully rotated arm.

Stabilization: The free hand, as with the test of the inferior division, is placed on the back in order to prevent body rotation.

Patient: Pushes the arm backwards (dorsally) as hard as possible.

Examiner: Resists in a downward (anterior) direction to take the arm out of extension.

As with the inferior division, the trapezius muscle does not attach to the humerus. Therefore, in order to determine weakness, one must visually observe for scapular movement during the test. Fixation of the medial border of the scapula is crucial for the test. When the arm and the medial border of the scapula move together, the middle trapezius is deemed weak. However, when the medial border remains in place, but the tested arm moves anteriorly, weakness of the posterior fixators of the shoulder, mainly the posterior deltoid, is implied.

The test can also be made in the supine position where stabilization of the patient is better but where palpation of the scapula is either more difficult or almost impossible. The weight of the body against the table surface in this position tends to block scapular movement and may cause false negative findings.

Stabilization of the anterior aspect of the shoulder on the tested side is necessary when the patient is in a sitting or standing position.

Test errors, precautions: As with the inferior division, the test must be carried out very specifically, as the testing lever is long compared to the strength of the muscle in the average patient. With apparent weakness, it is best to evaluate the other shoulder joint extensors and the lower trapezius as well.

Myofascial syndrome

Stretch test: Is not very clinically significant as trigger points frequently develop due to muscle fatigue rather than as a consequence of prolonged stretching. It is common to find contracted pectoralis muscles that reflexively inhibit the trapezius, causing the development of trigger points. In chronic situations a hyperkyphosis may develop.

Frequently found associated disorders

Structurally, recurring rib dysfunction occurs and, in rare cases, may be associated with microfixations of the mid-dorsals.

Leaf (1996) describes a situation whereby a compensatory weakening of the middle trapezius may be used to demonstrate a general inhibition pattern of the trunk extensors when in the presence of hyper-tonic plantar foot muscles. The middle trapezius is tested with the patient seated and then standing. When the trapezius tests strong when seated, but weak upon standing, it is assumed that a widespread inhibition of the back extensors exists.

Compression weakness: Lesions involving the base of the skull, the occipital condyles, atlas, the C3 root and the jugular foramen.

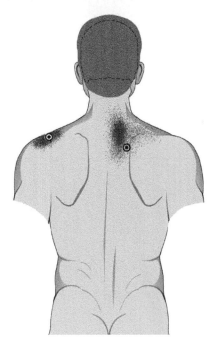

Trigger points and referred pain pattern.
Note: The lateral trigger point seen in the
illustration on the left is shown on the left in
this figure, the medial one on the right.

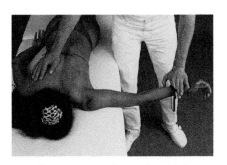

Test of the horizontal fibres. The stabilizing
hand may be placed on the scapula on
the tested side in order to better register
movement, however, rotational stabilization is
made less secure

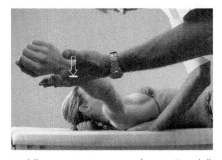

Middle trapezius test according to Beardall

M. trapezius,
horizontal and
ascending fibres

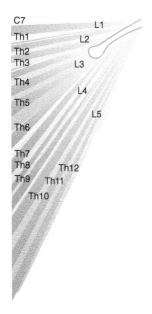

Motor function innervation: Spinal accessory
nerve, anterior branches of the cervical nerves
2, 3, 4
Visceroparietal segment (TS line): T7
Organ: Spleen
Nutrients: Vitamin C, calcium
Meridian: Spleen
Rib pump zone: Intercostal space,
costotransverse joint 7, 11

Spondylogenic reflex zones for the horizontal
and ascending fibres of the trapezius

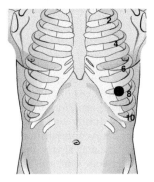

NL anterior

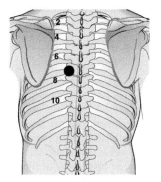

NL posterior

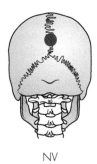

NV

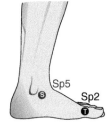

Anatomy

Origin: From the external occipital protuberance, the middle third of the superior nuchal line, the nuchal ligament and the C7 spinous process.

Course: The superior fibres descend almost vertically and then progress anteriorly towards the lateral third of the clavicle. The more inferior fibres run almost horizontally. It lies superficial to and covers the levator scapulae and rhomboid muscles.

Insertion: At the lateral third of the clavicle and the acromion process of the scapula, as well as the lateral, superior margin the scapular spine.

Action

It elevates the shoulder and rotates the scapula so that the glenoid cavity moves superiorly. When the scapula is fixed, a lateral flexion and extension of both the head and cervical spine occurs. It assists in rotation of the head to the opposite side, as well.

Signs of weakness: An abnormally low shoulder when standing and with bilateral weakness the head position is anterior to the midline of the shoulders.

Test

Position: The patient should be seated at a level that permits the examiner's trunk to be well above the head of the patient. This position is better suited for pulling the head superiorly during the test. Ideally, the examiner stands opposite the side being tested. One may also be take a position on the same side, as is illustrated, but the resistance vector must be strictly followed. The patient lifts the shoulder as high as possible and inclines the head such that the ear is brought close to the elevated shoulder. The ear to shoulder position will automatically rotate the head slightly so that the nose points about 15° to the side opposite the test. If this is not noted, further rotation of the head should be made.

Test contact: With the flat of the hand, a broad contact is made just above the ear, on the parietal bone of the tested side.

Stabilization: The other, free hand is placed on the elevated shoulder. The hands of the examiner will be almost touching one another when the head and shoulder are correctly positioned.

Patient: Attempts to maintain the start position.

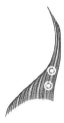

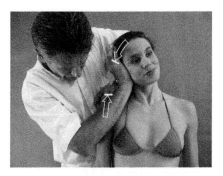

Upper trapezius test

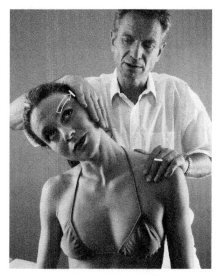

PIR of the upper trapezius with sustained inspiration and gentle contraction

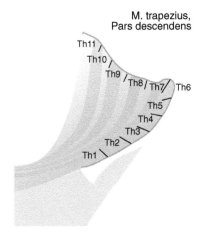

Alternative testing position

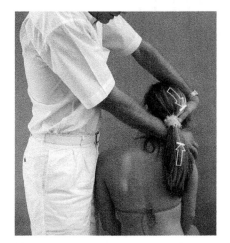

**M. trapezius,
Pars descendens**

Th11
Th10
Th9
Th8 Th7 Th6
Th5
Th4
Th3
Th2
Th1

Spondylogenic reflex zones for the upper trapezius

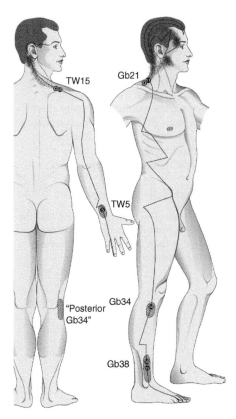

TW15   Gb21

TW5

"Posterior Gb34"   Gb34

Gb38

Trigger points, referred pain pattern and effective distal points

Examiner: The examiner should be positioned so that it is possible to pull the head superiorly. Thereafter, the main resistance on the head is directed so as to separate the ear from the shoulder. Due to the short levers, it is important that the test vector is strictly adhered to.

Alternatively, in a procedure that is more difficult, the examiner can stand on the same side of the tested muscle. Here the patient position should be slightly higher than that of the examiner. The hands, like the position above, are placed between the patient's head and shoulder. While the testing vectors are the same, the position of the examiner, in order to maintain the optimal direction of resistance, is at a disadvantage. In this instance, the examiner's testing hand should be below the level of the head of the patient so that resistance pressure can be made in a superior (cranial) direction. The hand on the shoulder will now pull, rather than push downward.

Test errors, precautions: Too little elevation of the shoulder and lack of rotation of the head so that the ear is placed anterior to the midline of the shoulder. With less than an optimum positioning, the examiner is easily at a disadvantage. Precise resistance vectors will be difficult to maintain and the patient will be able to bring other synergistic muscles into play.

Myofascial syndrome

Stretch test: The patient is seated and the shoulder is held down by the examiner. The head is then laterally flexed to the opposite side and then anteriorly.

Stretch can also be performed with the patient supine. The shoulder is manually depressed by the examiner, the head inclined laterally to the opposite side and slightly rotated to the side of stretch.

PIR: From the stretch position and with a sustained inspiration, the patient gradually brings the head back to a neutral, erect position. The relaxation phase follows with the patient slowly breathing out as the examiner gently returns the head to the start position and then slightly beyond to increase the stretching effect a bit more.

Frequently found associated disorders

Together with the levator scapulae the upper trapezius muscles harbour more trigger points than any other muscles of the body. When the two are compared, the upper trapezius is, without question, a refuge for the greater number of trigger points. Consequently, it is known as the quintessential 'psychosomatic stress muscle'.

According to Leaf (1996), hypertonicity of the plantar foot muscles will lead to inhibition of all spinal extensor muscles, including the three divisions of the trapezius muscle. A description of this inhibitory relationship and test is found in the middle trapezius chapter.

Compression weakness: Mechanical lesions of the third and fourth cervical vertebrae and the base of the skull. Restrictions of the temporo-occipital sutures or occipitoatlantal articulations might negatively affect the jugular foramen and compromise the spinal accessory nerve.

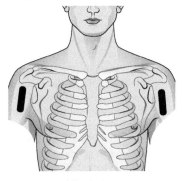

NL anterior

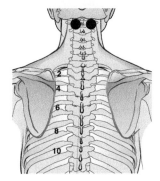

NL posterior

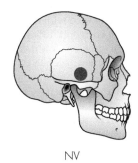

NV

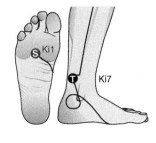

Motor function innervation: Spinal accessory nerve (XI), anterior branches of the cervical nerves 2, 3, 4
Organ: Eye, ear
Nutrients: Vitamins A, B2, B3, B-complex, bioflavonoides, PUFA, Ca
Meridian: Kidney

Anatomy

Origin: M. triceps brachii:
Long head: At the infraglenoidal tubercle of the scapula.

Lateral head: At the lateral and posterior aspect of the proximal half of the humerus.

Medial head: Below the sulcus of the radial nerve on the distal two-thirds of the medial and dorsal surface of the humerus.

M. anconeus: The origin is on the dorsal surface of the lateral epicondyle of the humerus.

Course: The fibres of the triceps brachii run mainly from superior to inferior but radiate more diagonally as they progress distally.

Insertion: M. triceps brachii: On the posterior surface of the olecranon and the antebrachial fascia.

M. anconeus: On the lateral side of the olecranon and at the proximal quarter of the dorsal surface of the ulna.

Action

Both muscles, overall, extend the elbow joint. The long head of the triceps also assists in adduction and extension of the humerus.

Although the function of the anconeus is not considered important in humans anymore, it resembles in action the extensor function of the lateral head of the triceps.

An accessory function of the anconeus may be to aid in pulling the joint capsule taught during full extension of the elbow to keep it from being pinched by the olecranon.

Signs of weakness: Flexion of the arm at the elbow.

Test

Function at the elbow

Position: The elbow is flexed to about 80° and the forearm is placed in a neutral position with respect to pronation and supination. The thumb will point up so that the radial bone is above the ulnar bone. This is a global test of all three heads.

According to Beardall (1982) the three heads may be differentiated from one another by changing the rotation of the forearm. Full supination of the forearm will test the lateral head, the neutral, 'thumb up' position will test the long head and with the forearm pronated the medial head is isolated. Whether these forearm nuances are sufficient to isolate the various heads of the triceps is still under discussion.

Again according to Beardall, the anconeus can be tested with the forearm in supination and with only 10° of flexion at the elbow. Nevertheless, it is dubious at best whether any test will be very specific for the anconeus.

Test contact: On the distal forearm. The area will be related to the degree of rotation used. The stabilizing hand is placed anteriorly over the anticubital fold of the elbow.

Patient: Extends the elbow as hard as possible.

Examiner: Resists trying to flex the elbow. If weakness is noted, resistance should follow the arc of motion of the forearm as it flexes.

Function at the shoulder (long head)

Position: Tested with the elbow flexed to about 90° and the humerus extended at the shoulder. Flexion of the elbow elongates the muscle over the elbow joint and contracts the muscle over the shoulder joint. Because the muscle acts on two joints, the position allows maximal contractile force to be directed at the posterior shoulder. The elbow should be abducted slightly from the trunk in order to better align the origin and insertion.

Test contact: The distal, posterior aspect of the humerus, close to the elbow.

Stabilization: On the anterior shoulder on the tested side.

Patient: Pulls the elbow backwards as hard as possible against the examiner's resistance.

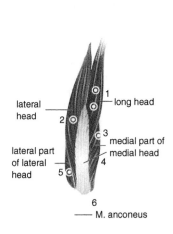

lateral head

1 — long head

2

lateral part of lateral head

3 — medial part of medial head

4

5

6 — M. anconeus

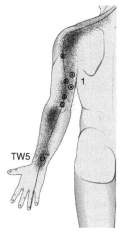

Trigger points in the long head

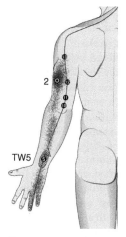

Trigger point in the lateral head

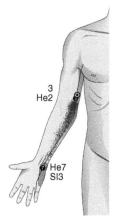

Trigger point in the medial margin of the medial head

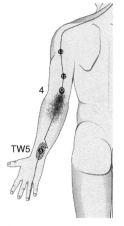

Trigger point deep in the medial head

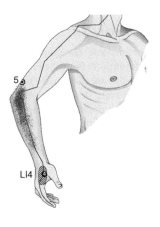

Trigger point in the lateral margin of the medial head

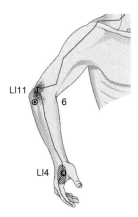

Trigger point in the anconeus

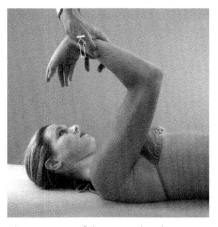

Alternative test of the triceps brachii

Alternative general test at the elbow for all heads

Position: The patient is supine, the elbow flexed to 90° and the upper arm flexed at the shoulder about 30–40°.

Test contact: To the patient's distal forearm.

Patient: Pushes the forearm into extension. For the supine patient this will be diagonally upwards (Portelli, oral information). The test is dependent upon good stabilization by the shoulder flexors in order to maintain fixation of the joint.

Test errors, precautions: Unless dealing with an extremely strong individual, the elbow should not be flexed by more than 90°. The arm must be optimally stabilized during the test and, where indicated, the shoulder must remain in a stable position.

Myofascial syndrome

Stretch test: The patient may be seated or lie supine. Both the elbow and the shoulder are maximally flexed.

Difficulty or an inability in elevating the arm with the elbow in flexion, whereas the patient cannot lift the forearm to the ear, is an indication of shortening, tension or trigger points in the long head of the triceps.

PIR: Starting from the stretch position and with a sustained inspiration, the examiner provides gentle resistance while the patient is instructed to slowly contract the triceps by slowly extending the elbow and shoulder at the same time. This is done by moving the elbow downwards and the hand upwards.

While the patient breathes out, the examiner returns the limb to the stretch position and then slightly beyond to further increase the elongation of the muscle.

Cause for compression: Trigger points in the lateral head can lead to irritation of the radial nerve in the area of the sulcus of the radius. Symptoms may include dysaesthesia (an unpleasant or abnormal sense of touch not necessarily associated with pain) in the area of the dorsal forearm and/or the back of the hand caused by the superficial branch. The deep group of forearm extensors can show weakness and dysfunction.

Frequently found associated disorders

Trigger points in the area of the anconeus can imitate the pain of tennis elbow (lateral epicondylitis). Tennis elbow can often be treated with dry needling of the trigger point in the area of the junction of the distal fibres of the lateral head of the triceps and the triceps tendon. This area is close to the anconeus muscle.

The more internal fibres of the medial head can develop trigger points and imitate golfer's elbow (medial epicondylitis). It can also occur together with lateral epicondylitis. Normally only with the use of a combined treatment is it possible to alleviate both conditions. A needling of the trigger points and local treatment for the periosteal irritation in the area of the epicondyle is usually required.

Compression weakness: The triceps brachii weakens with lesions of the root C7 (disc C6/7). Also scalenus, costoclavicular, and pectoralis minor syndromes may affect the triceps.

Motor function innervation: Radial nerve, C6, C7, C8, T1
Rib pump zone: Intercostal space, costotransverse joint 2, 10
Organ: Pancreas
Nutrients: Vitamins A, B3, Zn, Se, Cr, Mg, enzymes, PUFA
Meridian: Spleen (pancreas)

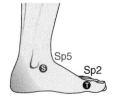

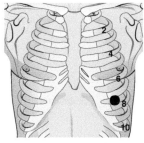

NL anterior

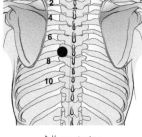

NL posterior

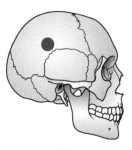

NV

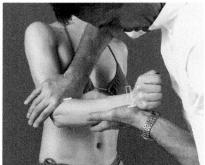

Test of the long head

Test of the medial head

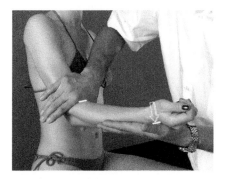

Test of the lateral head

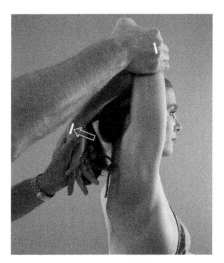

PIR: contraction phase with inspiration

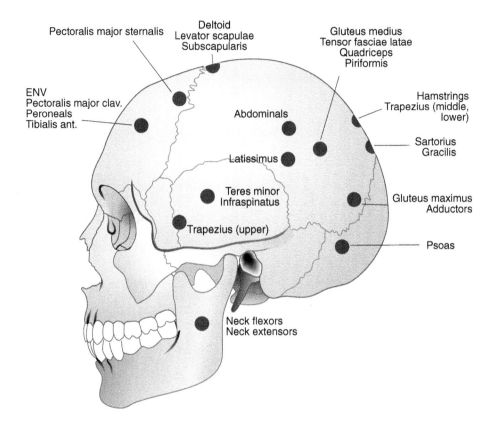

Pectoralis major sternalis

Deltoid
Levator scapulae
Subscapularis

Gluteus medius
Tensor fasciae latae
Quadriceps
Piriformis

ENV
Pectoralis major clav.
Peroneals
Tibialis ant.

Abdominals

Hamstrings
Trapezius (middle, lower)

Sartorius
Gracilis

Latissimus

Teres minor
Infraspinatus

Gluteus maximus
Adductors

Trapezius (upper)

Psoas

Neck flexors
Neck extensors

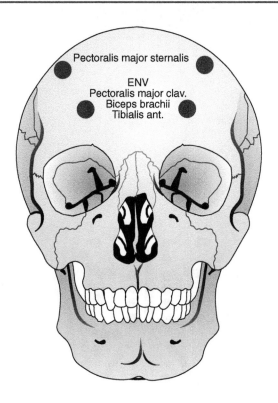

Pectoralis major sternalis

ENV
Pectoralis major clav.
Biceps brachii
Tibialis ant.

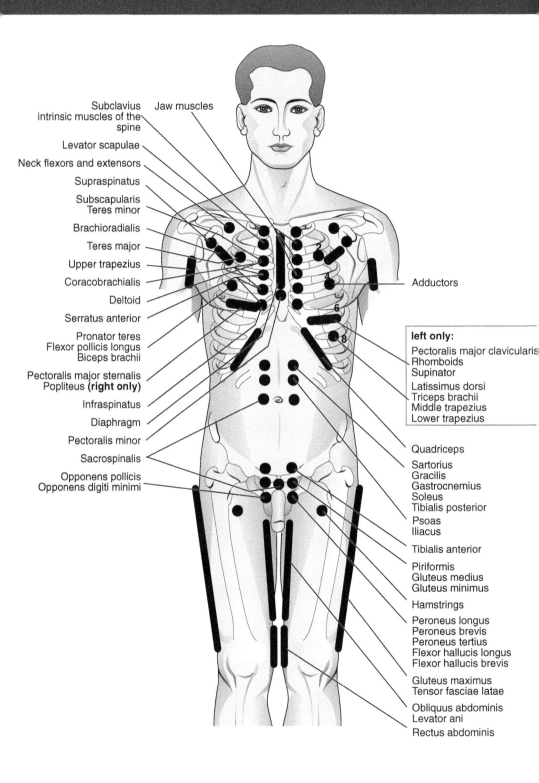

Subclavius
intrinsic muscles of the
spine
Jaw muscles
Levator scapulae
Neck flexors and extensors
Supraspinatus
Subscapularis
Teres minor
Brachioradialis
Teres major
Upper trapezius
Coracobrachialis
Deltoid
Serratus anterior
Pronator teres
Flexor pollicis longus
Biceps brachii
Pectoralis major sternalis
Popliteus (right only)
Infraspinatus
Diaphragm
Pectoralis minor
Sacrospinalis
Opponens pollicis
Opponens digiti minimi

Adductors

left only:
Pectoralis major clavicularis
Rhomboids
Supinator
Latissimus dorsi
Triceps brachii
Middle trapezius
Lower trapezius

Quadriceps
Sartorius
Gracilis
Gastrocnemius
Soleus
Tibialis posterior
Psoas
Iliacus

Tibialis anterior

Piriformis
Gluteus medius
Gluteus minimus

Hamstrings

Peroneus longus
Peroneus brevis
Peroneus tertius
Flexor hallucis longus
Flexor hallucis brevis

Gluteus maximus
Tensor fasciae latae

Obliquus abdominis
Levator ani

Rectus abdominis

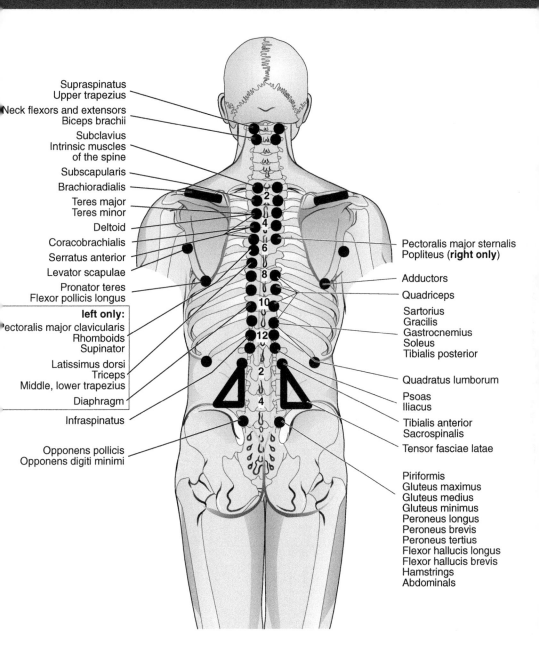

Supraspinatus
Upper trapezius
Neck flexors and extensors
Biceps brachii
Subclavius
Intrinsic muscles
of the spine
Subscapularis
Brachioradialis
Teres major
Teres minor
Deltoid
Coracobrachialis
Serratus anterior
Levator scapulae
Pronator teres
Flexor pollicis longus

left only:
Pectoralis major clavicularis
Rhomboids
Supinator
Latissimus dorsi
Triceps
Middle, lower trapezius
Diaphragm
Infraspinatus

Opponens pollicis
Opponens digiti minimi

Pectoralis major sternalis
Popliteus (**right only**)

Adductors
Quadriceps

Sartorius
Gracilis
Gastrocnemius
Soleus
Tibialis posterior

Quadratus lumborum

Psoas
Iliacus

Tibialis anterior
Sacrospinalis

Tensor fasciae latae

Piriformis
Gluteus maximus
Gluteus medius
Gluteus minimus
Peroneus longus
Peroneus brevis
Peroneus tertius
Flexor hallucis longus
Flexor hallucis brevis
Hamstrings
Abdominals

	Phylogenetic extensors (posterior) functional extensors	Phylogenetic flexors (anterior) functional flexors
C3		
	Scalenus syndrome	Scalenus syndrome
	Costoclavicular syndrome	
	Suprascapularis nerve syndrome	
C4	Coracopectoral syndrome	
	Sulcus n. radialis syndrome	
	Synd. of. lat. axillary space · Supinator syndrome	
		Costoclavicular syndrome
		Coracopectoral syndrome
C5		Pronator teres syndrome
		Carpal tunnel syndrome
C6		Ulnar sulcus syndrome
		Ulnar tunnel syndrome
C7		
C8		
Th1		

Cervical branches: superior trapezius (beside nerve XI)

Dorsal scapular nerve: rhomboids, levator scapulae

Suprascapular nerve: supraspinatus and infraspinatus

Long thoracic nerve: serratus anterior

Subscapular nerve: subscapularis, teres major

Axillary nerve: deltoideus, teres minor

Thoracodorsal nerve: latissimus dorsi

Radial nerve: triceps brachii

Radial nerve: brachioradialis

Radial nerve: extensor carpi radialis (C5–C8), supinator (C5–C7)

Radial nerve: extensor digitorum, extensor carpi ulnaris, abductor pollicis longus

Subclavian nerve: subclavius

Musculocutaneous nerve: biceps brachii, brachialis, coracobrachialis

Lateral pectoral nerve: pectoralis major clavicularis

Medial pectoral nerve: pectoralis major sternalis, pectoralis minor

Median nerve: flexor carpi radialis (C6–C8), pronator teres (C6, C7)

Median nerve: flexor digitalis superficialis, flexor pollicis longus, palmaris longus

Median nerve: flexor digitalis profundus (2nd and 3rd fingers), pronator quadratus, lumbricals I and II

Median nerve: opponens pollicis, abductor pollicis brevis

Ulnar nerve: flexor carpi ulnaris, flexor digitorum profundus (4th and 5th fingers)

Ulnar nerve: opponens digiti minimi, lumbricals II and IV

Ulnar nerve: dorsal and palmar interosseus muscles, lumbricals II and IV, adductor pollicis, flexor digiti minimi

Nerves of the lumbosacral plexus and nerve bottlenecks

Anterior muscle groups
Posterior muscle groups
L1
L2
L3
L4
L5
S1
S2
S3
Lumbar plexus: psoas
Iliopsoas-inguinal syndrome
Obturator syndrome
Femoral nerve: iliacus
Femoral nerve: pectineus
Femoral nerve: quadriceps, sartorius
Anterior obturator nerve: adductor brevis, longus and magnus; gracilis
Fibularis syndrome
Fibular nerve deep branch: tibialis anterior
Fibular nerve deep branch: extensor hallucis longus, extensor digitorum longus; peroneus tertius
Posterior obturator nerve: obturator externus, adductor magnus
Piriformis syndrome
Iliolumbal ligament syndrome
Fibularis syndrome
Piriform nerve: piriformis muscle
Superior gluteal nerve: gluteus medius and minimus, tensor fasciae latae
Inferior gluteal nerve: gluteus maximus
Sciatic nerve: biceps femoris, semimembranosus, semitendinosus
Fibular nerve, superficial branch: peroneus longus and brevis
Tibial nerve: popliteus
Popliteus syndrome
Tibial nerve: soleus, posterior tibialis, flexor digitorum longus, flexor hallucis longus
Tarsal tunnel syndrome
Tibial nerve: gastrocnemius
Tibial nerve (medial plantar): flexor hallucis brevis, flexor digitorum brevis
Tibial nerve (lateral plantar): quadratus plantae, adductor hallucis

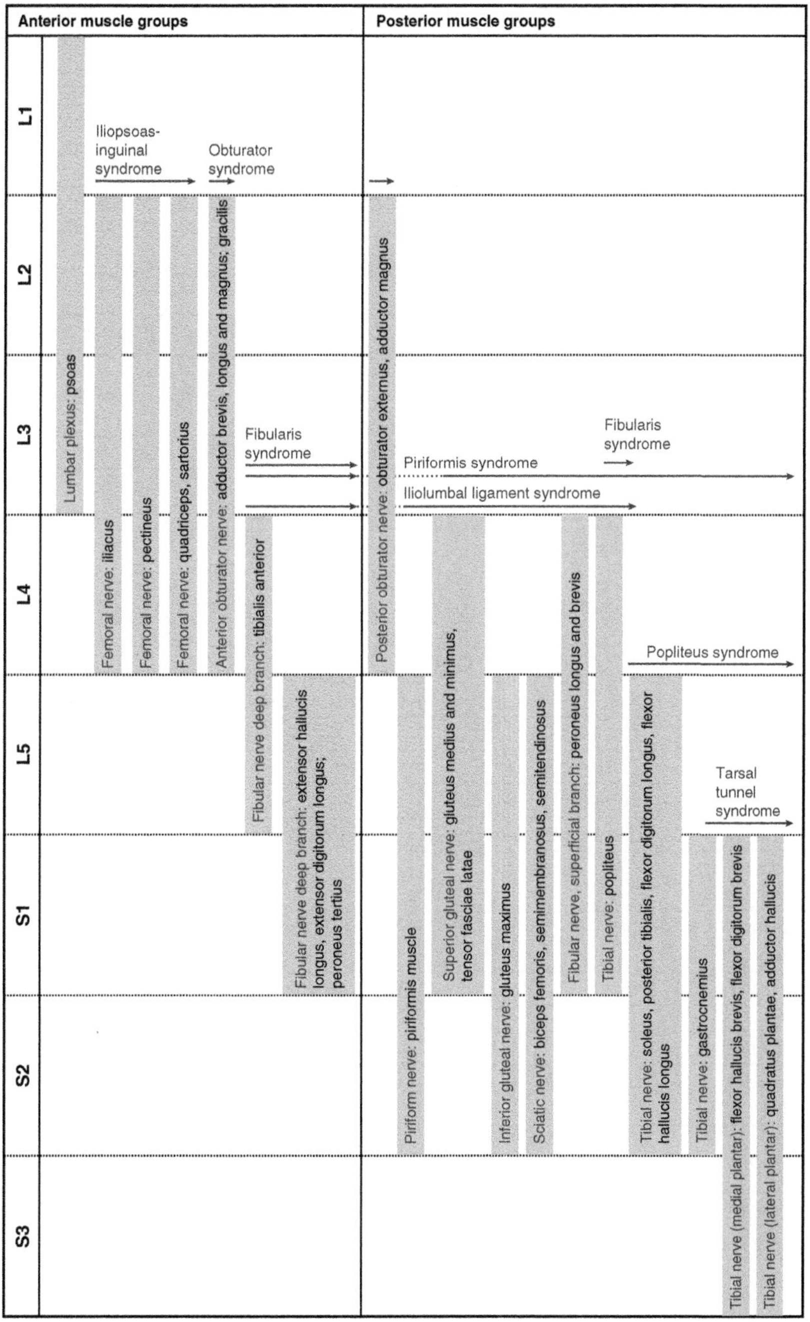

Muscles – organ (meridian) – relation to nutrients

Muscle	Organ (Meridian)	Orthomolecular Substances
Abdominal muscles	Small intestine (SI)	Vit. E, enzymes, betain-HCl, eubiotics, l-glutamine
Adductors	Gonads (Pe)	Vit. A, B3, C, E, PUFA, Zn, Se, Mg
Biceps brachii	Stomach (St)	Phosphatase
Coracobrachialis	Lung (Lu)	Vit. C, E, beta-carotene, Se, N-acetyl-cystein
Deltoid	Lung (Lu)	Vit. C, E, beta-carotene, Se, N-acetyl-cystein
Diaghragm	Conception vessel (CV)	
Extensors, flexors of the wrist	Stomach (St)	Phosphatase, Fe, Vit. B5, PUFA
Flex. hallucis (long., brev.)	Tarsal tunnel	Ca, Mg, Fe, phosphatase, Vit. B5, PUFA
Gastrocnemius	Adrenal (Pe)	Vit. B3, B5, B6, B9, B12, C, tyrosine, adrenal extract
Gluteus maximus	Gonads (Pe)	Vit. A, B3, C, E, PUFA, Zn, Se, Mg
Gluteus medius/ minimus	Gonads (Pe)	Vit. A, B3, C, E, PUFA, Zn, Se, Mg
Gracilis	Adrenal (Pe)	Vit. B3, B5, B6, B9, B12, C, tyrosine, adrenal extract
Hamstrings	Rectum (LI)	Vit. E, Ca, Mg, l-glutamine
Ileocecal valve (ICV)		Ca, Mg, eubiotics, chlorophyll
Infraspinatus	Thymus (TW)	Se, Zn, Cu, antioxidants, immunstim. phytotherapeutics
Latissimus dorsi	Pancreas (Sp)	Vit. A, B3, Zn, Se, Cr, Mg, enzymes, PUFA
Levator scapulae	Parathyroid (Lu)	Ca, Mg, Vit. D
Neck extensors	Paranasal sinuses (St)	Vit. B3, B6, iodine
Neck flexors	Paranasal sinuses (St)	Vit. B3, B6, iodine
Opponens pol.- digiti min.	Carpal tunnel (St)	Vit. B6, B5, Fe, PUFA, phosphatase
Pectoralis major clavicularis	Stomach (St)	Betain-HCl, buffer substances, vit. B1, B12, Zn
Pectoralis major sternalis	Liver (Li)	Vit. A, B-compl., l-glutathione, NAC, carduus marianus
Pectoralis minor		Antioxidants, low dose Vit. A
Peroneus long./ brev./tert.	Bladder (Bl)	Vit. A, B1, B-complex, K
Piriformis	Gonads (Pe)	Vit. A, B3, C, E, PUFA, Zn, Se, Mg
Popliteus	Gall bladder (Gb)	Vit. A, beta-carotene
Pronator teres	Stomach (St)	Ca, Mg, Fe, phosphatase, Vit. B5, PUFA
Psoas, Iliopsoas	Kidney (Ki)	Vit. A, E
Quadratus lumborum	Appendix (LI)	Vit. A, Vit. E, eubiotics
Quadriceps	Small intestine (SI)	Ca, vit D, B-complex, CoQ10, eubiotics
Rhomboids	Liver (Li)	Vit. A, C, antioxidants
Sacrospinalis	Bladder (Bl)	Vit. A, E, C, Ca

Muscle	Organ (Meridian)	Orthomolecular Substances
Sartorius	Adrenal (Pe)	Vit. B3, B5, B6, B9, B12, C, tyrosine, adrenal extract
Serratus anterior	Lung (Lu)	Vit. C, E, beta-carotene, Se, N-acetyl-cystein
Soleus	Adrenal (Pe)	
Sternocleidomastoid	Paranasal sinuses (Ma)	Vit. B3, B6, iodine
Subclavius		Mg
Subscapularis	Heart (He)	Vit. B2, B3, E, Mg, l-carnitine
Supinator	Stomach (St)	Ca, Mg, Fe, phosphatase, Vit. B5, PUFA
Supraspinatus	Brain (GV)	PUFA, phosphatidyl-choline, antioxidants
Tensor fascia latae	Large intestine (LI)	Eubiotics, l-glutamine, Fe
Teres major	Spine (GV)	
Teres minor	Thyroid (TW)	Iode, Se, Zn, Mn, Vit. A, B-compl., tyrosine
Tibialis anterior	Bladder (Bl)	Vit. A, B1, B-complex, potassium
Tibialis posterior	Adrenal (Pe)	Vit. B3, B5, B6, B9, B12, C, tyrosine, adrenal extract
Trapezius – upper	Eye, ear (Ki)	Vit. A, B2, B3, B-compl., bioflavonoids, PUFA, Ca
Trapezius – lower, mid	Spleen (Sp)	Vit. C, Ca
Triceps brachii	Pancreas (Sp)	Vit. A, B3, Zn, Se, Cr, Mg, enzymes, PUFA

Angermaier, U.S., 2006. Studie zur Sedationsfähigkeit von Magneten. Applied Kinesiology 1 (1).

Beardall, A.G., 1980. Clinical Kinesiology, Vol. I: Muscles of the Low Back and Abdomen. Human Biodynamics, Portland, OR.

Beardall, A.G., 1981. Clinical Kinesiology, Vol. II: Muscles of the Pelvis and Thigh. Human Biodynamics, Portland, OR.

Beardall, A.G., 1983. Clinical Kinesiology, Vol. IV: Muscles of the Upper Extremities, Forearm and Hand. Human Biodynamics, Portland, OR.

Beardall, A.G., 1985. Clinical Kinesiology, Vol. V: Muscles of the Lower Extremities, Calf and Foot. Human Biodynamics, Portland, OR.

Bergsmann, O., Bergsmann, R., 1997. Projektionssyndrome. Facultas, Vienna.

Carpenter, S., Hoffman, J., Mendel, R., 1977. An investigation into the effects of organ irritation on muscle strength and spinal mobility. Bull Eur Chiropr Union 25 (2), 42–60.

Chaitow, L., 1988. Soft-Tissue Manipulation. Thorsons, Wellingborough.

Chapman, F., 1936. An Endocrine Interpretation of Chapman's Reflexes. Owens.

Dvořák, J., Dvořák, V., 1991. Manuelle Medizin, Diagnostik. Thieme, Stuttgart.

Frick, H., Leonhardt, H., Stark, D., 1992a. Allgemeine Anatomie, Spezielle Anatomie 1. Thieme, Stuttgart.

Frick, H., Leonhardt, H., Stark, D., 1992b. Spezielle Anatomie 2. Thieme, Stuttgart.

Garten, H., 2012. Applied Kinesiology: Muskelfunktion, Dysfunktion, Therapie, second ed. Urban und Fischer, München.

Garten, H., Weiss, G., 2007. Sytemische Störungen, Problemfälle lösen mit Applied Kinesiology. Urban und Fischer, München.

Gerz, W., 2000. Applied Kinesiology in der Naturheilkundlichen Praxis. AKSE-Verlag, Wörthsee.

Goodheart, G.J., 1964. Applied Kinesiology. 20567 Mack Ave., Grosspoint, MI, 48236-1655. USA, privately published.

Goodheart, G.J., 1965. Applied Kinesiology 1965 Workshop Procedure Manual, second ed. 20567 Mack Ave., Grosspoint, MI, 48236-1655, USA, privately published.

Goodheart, G.J., 1966. Chinese lessons for chiropractic. Chiro Econ 8 (5).

Goodheart, G.J., 1970. Applied Kinesiology 1970 Workshop Procedure Manual, seventh ed. 20567 Mack Ave., Grosspoint, MI, 48236-1655, USA, privately published.

Goodheart, G.J., 1971. Applied Kinesiology 1971 Workshop Procedure Manual, eighth ed. 20567 Mack Ave., Grosspoint, MI, 48236-1655, USA, privately published.

Goodheart, G.J., 1976. Applied Kinesiology 1976 Workshop Procedure Manual, twelfth ed. 20567 Mack Ave., Grosspoint, MI, 48236-1655, USA, privately published.

Goodheart, G.J., 1979. Applied Kinesiology 1979 Workshop Procedure Manual, fifteenth ed. 20567 Mack Ave., Grosspoint, MI, 48236-1655, USA, privately.

Hack, G.D., Koritzer, R.T., Robinson, W.L., et al., 1995. Anatomic relation between the rectus capitis posterior minor muscle and the dura mater. Spine 20 (23), 2484–2486.

Janda, V., 1994. Manuelle Muskelfunktionsdiagnostik. Ullstein-Mosby, Berlin.

Jones, L.H., 1981. Strain and Counterstrain. American Academy of Osteopathy, Newark.

Kendall, H.O., Kendall, F.P., 1952. Functional Muscle Testing. Physical Medicine and General Practice, Chapt. XII. Paul B. Hoeber, New York.

Kendall, F., Kendall, E., 1983. Muscle-testing and Function. Williams and Wilkins, Baltimore.

Leaf, D., 1979. A Validation Study on the Effects of Music on the Muscle Strength of the Body. Proceedings of Summer Meeting, Detroit, International College of Applied Kinesiology.

Leaf, D., 1996. Applied Kinesiology Flowchart Manual. MoJo-Enterprise, Samoset, MA.

Lewit, K., 1992. Manuelle Medizin. Johann Ambrosius Barth, Leipzig.

Lines, D.H., McMillan, A.J., Spehr, G.J., 1990. Effects of soft tissue technique and Chapman's neurolymphatic reflex stimulation on respiratory function. Journal of the Australian Chiropractors' Association 20, 17–22.

Lovett, R.W., Martin, E.G., 1916. Certain aspects of infantile paralysis with a description of a method of muscle testing. JAMA 66 (10).

Mense, S., 2003. The pathogenesis of muscle pain. Curr Pain Headache Rep 7 (6), 419–425.

Mense, S., 2004. Neurobiological basis for the use of botulinum toxin in pain therapy. J Neurol 251 (Suppl. 1), I1–7.

Mitchell, F.L.J., 1995. The Muscle Energy Manual. MET Press, East Lansing, Michigan.

Palastanga, N., Field, D., Soames, R., 1989. Anatomy and Human Movement: Structure and Function. Butterworth-Heinemann, Oxford.

Patten, J., 1998. Neurologische Differentialdiagnose. Springer, Berlin.

Rauch, E., 1994. Lehrbuch der Diagnostik und Therapie nach F.X.Mayr. Haug, Heidelberg.

Schiebler, T.H., Schmidt, W., Zilles, K., 1999. Anatomie, Zytologie, Histologie, Entwicklungsgeschichte, Makroskopische und Mikroskopische Anatomie des Menschen. Springer, Berlin.

Schmitt, W.H., Yanuck, S.F., 1999. Expanding the neurological examination using functional neurological assessment part II. Int Neurosci 97, 77–108.

Schupp, W., 1993. Funktionslehre in der Kieferorthopädie. Fachdienst der Kieferorthopäden, Bergisch Gladbach.

Siebert, G.K., 1995. Atlas der Zahnärztlichen Funktionsdiagnostik. Hanser, München.

Sutter, M., 1975. Wesen, Klinik und Bedeutung Spondylogener Reflexsyndrome. Schweiz Rdsch Med Prax 64 (42), 1351–1357.

Travell, J.G., Simons, D.G., 1983. Myofascial Pain and Dysfunction. Williams & Wilkins, Baltimore.

Travell, J.G., Simons, D.G., 1992. Myofascial Pain and Dysfunction. Williams and Wilkins, Baltimore.

Walther, D.S., 1981. Applied Kinesiology, Vol. I. Systems D.C., Pueblo, CO.

Walther, D.S., 1983. Applied Kinesiology, Vol II. Systems D.C., Pueblo, CO.

Walther, D.S., 2000. Applied Kinesiology, Synopsis. Systems D.C., Pueblo, CO.

Winkel, D., Vleeming, A., Fisher, S. (Eds.), 1985. Nichtoperative Orthopädie der Weichteile des Bewegungsapparates, Teil 2. Gustav Fischer, Stuttgart.

Page numbers followed by 'f' indicate figures, 't' indicate tables, and 'b' indicate boxes.

Index of Muscles by Region

Page numbers followed by 'f' indicate figures, 't' indicate tables, and 'b' indicate boxes.

Printed and bound by CPI Group (UK) Ltd, Croydon, CR0 4YY

03/10/2024

01040848-0017